OBESITY

OBESITY

Kathleen Y. Wolin, Sc.D., and
Jennifer M. Petrelli

Biographies of Disease
Julie K. Silver, M.D., Series Editor

GREENWOOD PRESS
An Imprint of ABC-CLIO, LLC

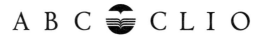

A B C CLIO

Santa Barbara, California • Denver, Colorado • Oxford, England

Library of Congress Cataloging-in-Publication Data

Wolin, Kathleen Y.
    Obesity / Kathleen Y. Wolin, Jennifer M. Petrelli.
        p. cm. – (Biographies of disease)
    Includes bibliographical references and index.
    ISBN 978-0-313-35275-1 (hard copy: alk. paper) — ISBN 978-0-313-
35276-8 (ebook) 1. Obesity—Popular works. I. Petrelli, Jennifer M.
II. Title.
    RC628.W57 2009
    616.3′98–dc22   2009016117

13   12   11   10   9   1   2   3   4   5

This book is also available on the World Wide Web as an eBook.
Visit www.abc-clio.com for details.

ABC-CLIO, LLC
130 Cremona Drive, Box 1911
Santa Barbara, California 93116-1911

This book is printed on acid-free paper (∞)

Manufactured in the United States of America

KW: To Dylan, Charlotte, and Sosa, whose patience for the time this project took away from them and ongoing support for my work is underacknowledged but never underappreciated.

JP: To Mariano, for giving up the dining room table for many months and providing levity, and to the memory of Dr. Eugenia "Jeanne" Calle, a stellar mentor and a dear friend.

Contents

Series Foreword

Every disease has a story to tell: about how it started long ago and began to disable or even take the lives of its innocent victims, about the way it hurts us, and about how we are trying to stop it. In this Biographies of Disease series, the authors tell the stories of the diseases that we have come to know and dread.

The stories of these diseases have all of the components that make for great literature. There is incredible drama played out in real-life scenes from the past, present, and future. You'll read about how men and women of science stumbled trying to save the lives of those they aimed to protect. Turn the pages and you'll also learn about the amazing success of those who fought for health and won, often saving thousands of lives in the process.

If you don't want to be a health professional or research scientist now, when you finish this book you may think differently. The men and women in this book are heroes who often risked their own lives to save or improve ours. This is the biography of a disease, but it is also the story of real people who made incredible sacrifices to stop it in its tracks.

Julie K. Silver, M.D.
Assistant Professor, Harvard Medical School
Department of Physical Medicine and Rehabilitation

Preface

Obesity holds a unique place in the public health and medical fields as it is both a risk factor for other health outcomes and a health outcome all its own. *Obesity* aims to provide a comprehensive look at both the causes of obesity as an outcome and the health risks that being overweight and obese pose.

HOW TO USE THIS BOOK

This book begins with a look back, which provides perspective as subsequent chapters look forward. Each chapter in this book aims to build on the knowledge foundation provided in the previous chapters. While chapters build upon each other, each provides sufficient information to be read individually without loss of comprehension. Balancing breadth and depth, this book is the perfect text to add to a library or personal reference collection. Readers will benefit from the clear review of obesity-related research that is combined with lay press coverage of the condition.

Chapter 1 begins with a review of the history of obesity. This provides a context for the work that follows and is a foundation for understanding much modern thought on the causes and consequences of obesity. Chapter 2 defines the problem. It both defines what obesity is in a current medical sense and outlines the magnitude of the obesity problem in adults and children. It also provides a summary of how obesity is measured. Chapter 3 outlines the causes of obesity, including both lifestyle and genetic factors. The chapter includes a brief overview of energy balance and nutritional composition. Chapter 4 provides a review of the research on the most common health outcomes associated with obesity. The reader will understand the myriad of complications associated with obesity and how obesity might increase the risk of those conditions. This chapter also reviews two ongoing scientific debates about the harms associated with obesity. Chapter 5 explains the current research on preventing and treating obesity. Similarities and differences in what is done to prevent versus treat obesity are discussed. Potential negative side effects of some approaches are also reviewed. Chapter 6 is an analysis of the costs associated with obesity, including costs to the individual and society. Chapter 7 highlights the future of obesity research and treatment in the United States. Two state-of-the-art research projects on obesity prevention and treatment are considered in detail. This chapter focuses on both national and international issues associated with overweight and obesity while highlighting the global impact of obesity. The chapter also reviews one of the hot topics related to obesity: the influence of marketing and media.

ACKNOWLEDGMENTS

We thank Julie Silver for the opportunity to participate in this wonderful book series. We also thank our research assistants, Jenna Goldhaber and Angela Tanner, whose work pulling research was immensely helpful.

Introduction

The obesity epidemic is an inescapable truth that confronts us on a daily basis via the latest statistics about the number of people in the United States who are categorized as obese, advertisements for diet products, or our own observations of the people around us. There is a great deal of cause for alarm because although it is known that being obese is generally bad for health, we are at the dawn of the understanding of how seriously and deeply obesity can impact so many aspects of health and disease processes. For example, we now know, due to rigorous scientific inquiry, that obesity increases not only the risk of death, heart disease, and diabetes but also the risk of developing certain cancers.

The number of obese children in the United States is on the rise. Pediatricians are diagnosing high cholesterol and type 2 diabetes in children, and these are illnesses that traditionally do not present until adulthood. The epidemic of obesity in children and young adults not only threatens their quality of life but also threatens to shorten their life span. Thus, effective ways to prevent and treat obesity in childhood and adolescence are urgently needed.

Obesity has been documented by scientists over the ages and depicted and glorified in artwork spanning thousands of years. Although in some cultures corpulence was celebrated as a sign of prosperity, even ancient scientists such as Hippocrates recognized the detrimental consequences of obesity to health.

Obesity impacts all sectors of society, but it disproportionately affects some minority groups, especially African Americans and the growing Hispanic population in the United States. In addition, obesity is often an outward sign of poverty because the food that is affordable and available to low-income people in their living environment is often energy dense and nutrient poor. Exacerbating this, low-income people often live in unsafe neighborhoods, and this discourages physical activity.

The causes of obesity have been debated extensively, but it seems to come down to the fact that in present-day society, people are moving less and eating more than they did 50 years ago. In short, the United States has undergone a nutrition transition. More daily tasks have been mechanized (e.g., motorized transportation), and we have moved from an agrarian economy to one that is more service oriented and urban centered. This shift not only demands less of our bodies in terms of physical activity but also results in a shift in eating patterns away from eating traditional local foods and foods prepared in the home and toward consumption of mass-produced, high-calorie processed foods. In addition, the food that is available is delivered in larger quantities and has a high calorie value. Globally, countries such as Brazil, Russia, India, and China, which have experienced rapid economic expansion, are in the midst of their own nutrition transition.

The influence of advertising and media on how we think and the purchases we make has been studied in relation to the obesity epidemic, largely focusing on children and young adults. Although research in this area continues to grow along with new interactive media technologies, it has been hypothesized that media (e.g., watching television, playing computer games) displaces physical activity and that food advertisements and marketing to children contribute to overweight and obesity in this population.

The epidemic of obesity and its concomitant complications threaten to overwhelm the health care system in the United States and foreign countries that continue to try to stem the tide of HIV and other infectious diseases. The cost of managing the epidemic, which many point out is preventable, is to the detriment of treating other illnesses and draws money needed for other sectors of society such as education. Indeed, the consequences of overweight and obesity, as experienced on a population level, are far reaching and ultimately can threaten the economic viability of a country. Disabilities and premature death due to obesity rob society of its most productive members, and the lost income in addition to the cost of treating the complications of obesity prolong the poverty cycle to the next generation.

There is no quick fix to the issues posed by obesity. Unfortunately, losing weight is not easy, and intervention studies that have been done have not demonstrated long-term maintenance of weight loss. There is cause for hope because a few ongoing studies that have addressed lifestyle issues have been successful. So far, the results demonstrate that it takes perseverance, dedication, and a change in mind-set to achieve successful long-term weight loss. We look forward to the results of novel interventions such as the Be Fit, Be Well intervention (discussed in Chapter 7) that is currently underway to address not just caloric intake but also lifestyle changes and goal setting for behavior change.

When lifestyle modifications and diet are not successful, physicians may recommend drug therapy for obese adult patients. There are currently only a few drugs that are approved by the U.S. Food and Drug Administration for the purpose of obesity treatment. These drugs act by altering chemical signals that trigger feelings of fullness (satiety) or by decreasing the amount of fat absorbed by the body. However, there are adverse side effects that may result from taking drugs for obesity treatment, including gastrointestinal distress. There are safety concerns about prescribing weight loss drugs to obese adolescents due to the lack of studies in this population and the fact that these drugs may interfere with the normal growth of a young person.

Weight-loss surgery is another increasingly popular option, fueled by media reports of celebrity surgery, for treating obesity in extremely obese patients. Although gastric bypass surgery and adjustable gastric banding have been demonstrated to be successful, surgery is not without risk and the potential for complication. In addition, weight-loss surgery is not a stand-alone option for treating the extremely obese patient. In order to achieve successful long-term weight loss, surgery must be combined with lifestyle changes.

Obesity provides a thorough review of the history, causes, complications, and treatments of obesity.

1

History of Obesity

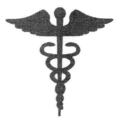

To say obesity has been around nearly as long as man isn't much of a stretch. Obese figures are depicted in Paleolithic artifacts found in Europe and the Middle East that date from 23,000 to 25,000 years ago. These depictions were likely deities of a bountiful harvest, and thus the depictions were done in an admiring fashion. Similarly corpulent figures, generally female, are found in Neolithic sites dating from 8000 to 5500 BCE. These depictions are often referred to as Mother Goddesses, and it is believed they were meant to invoke fertility (of people and plants) and bounty. Depictions of corpulent women continued well into the modern era in painting and sculpture (see Figure 1.1).

Moving into the Common Era, representations of obese women continue to appear. This is also when we start to see allusions to obesity in a negative light. Even before the age that we think of as representing the beginnings of scientific inquiry and scientific medicine (1500 CE and forward), obesity was seen as needing treatment. Ancient Egyptians found obesity objectionable. The Chinese used acupuncture to decrease appetite as a treatment for obesity. Ancient Tibetan medicine administered enemas and compresses to treat obesity. Indian medicine suggested treatment using organotherapy, specifically using testicular tissue. This was the time of Hippocrates, the father of modern

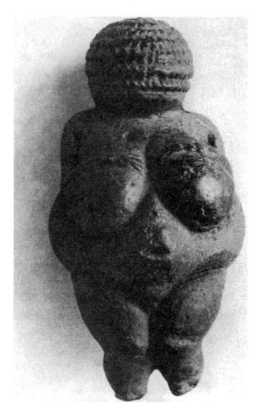

Figure 1.1. Venus von Willendorf [Photos.com].

medicine. He wrote of the risks associated with obesity, including infertility, sleep disruptions, and mortality. Galen, a prominent Roman physician living in the second century CE, identified moderate and immoderate obesity. These are likely parallels to our modern obese and morbidly obese classifications.

OBESITY IN SOCIETY

In more modern times, the diet and fitness movements have been tied to our country's puritanical religious history. The underlying philosophy behind much of the thinking throughout history has been that God intended the body to be perfect so any failure of that is the fault of the individual, who must assume responsibility for the state of his or her body and work for its vitality through diet and exercise (Whorton 1982, 5). The notion that disease could be prevented largely stemmed from the notion that epidemics were punishment from God for sin; thus, by leading a moral life, individuals could prevent the waves of disease that periodically wiped out large portions of society. The link between morality and obesity is not new and dates back several centuries. Remember, gluttony is one of the seven "deadly" sins. Medieval church leaders linked gluttony directly to eating and named the ways that man could commit gluttony:

- *Praepropere*: eating too soon
- *Laute*: eating too expensively (washedly)
- *Nimis*: eating too much
- *Ardenter*: eating too eagerly (burningly)
- *Studiose*: eating too daintily (keenly)
- *Forente*: eating wildly (boringly)

People believed that a fitter body would lead to improved mental abilities (and to some degree, modern research has supported this notion). But it is a slippery slope, as improved mental function implied to our forebears a stronger willpower, and it was willpower that one needed to protect oneself from the temptation of sin. It followed that an unfit body was the sign of a weak (and thus immoral) mind. This belief set has provided the foundation for much of the efforts to prevent and treat obesity in modern history—that educating people about how to have a fit body is sufficient to help them achieve one and that once they are of normal weight, individuals will find it so appealing that there will be minimal regression. As we'll see, this hasn't been the case by any stretch, and research has begun to look beyond the individual to the environmental and societal factors that may contribute to obesity.

As we think about how society viewed obesity, it is important to remember that what people thought was an appropriate response has changed dramatically over time. In the early 1800s there was little push to abstain entirely from anything (food or drink), but rather to pursue all things in moderation. Balance in the amount of food and exercise was considered by health promoters of the times, but relatively less emphasis was placed on the content or quality of either. Restriction in the form of fasting didn't become a common response to overweight until the turn of the century. Society in the 1800s was not amenable to notions of abstinence, so dieting seemed abnormal. Contrast that with the modern era, when surveys often find a large percentage of participants reporting they are actively monitoring their weight or taking steps, large and small, to maintain or lose weight.

While many of our contemporary images of dieting focus on women, it was not that way until the 20th century. Prior to then, the authors and famous examples of dieters were men. In fact, in the 1700s and 1800s dieting was a muscular, willful act—and thus one of middle-aged men. References at the time to women's dieting were an entirely different matter. Men at the time had noticed that women's weight seemed to change at puberty, marriage, pregnancy, and menopause and thus assumed the weight changes were about fluids, secretions, and sex—conflating the womb and the stomach. Observers of dieting history have commented that fat men are gluttons or monsters, while fat women are patients or freaks, unable to control themselves. As such, fat men inspire and fat women disgust. Fat men get diseases of the joints and hearts, while fat women get diseases of the glands or bad genes. History, and in many ways modern medicine, perceives male obesity as treatable to a much larger extent than female obesity.

While many famous diets came about as the "inventors" sought weight loss, not all diets were about being thin or thinner. Grahamites, whom we'll discuss in detail later, were interested in being vigorous. They thought gluttons were greedy and excessive and sought to live a life that spoke of charity by denying abundance and seeking resilience. Thinness wasn't the goal of the Graham diet—a wholesome, balanced appetite was. Grahamites resented the implication that they were freaks or ghosts. They claimed their diet, based on vegetables, fruit, and wheat bread, left them invigorated both physically and spiritually. It is in the Grahamites that we see the first large-scale documentation of weight by ordinary Americans. This was a group weighing themselves with regularity to help monitor their progress toward that vigorous goal.

WERE AMERICANS ALONE IN THEIR OBESITY?

Americans were outconsuming the rest of the world as early as the mid-1850s. At the time, this additional consumption, which was of meat and vegetables, meant that Americans were taller than their European and African counterparts by as much as three or four inches. Americans were accustomed to seeing more food on the table and eating more often. Modern eating research has found the more food placed in front of a person, the more he or she eats. American etiquette of the time dictated abundant meals and considered it rude to leave food on the plate. But Americans at the time were not largely obese, despite the consumption of huge quantities of food, especially meat. In fact, the world perceived the British as the corpulent people of the time, and Britain was the source of much of the writing on dieting and weight from the mid-18th to mid-19th century.

But the American situation was, in many ways, unique. Americans had access to cheap sugar—and a corresponding affection for sweet confections.

The first American cookbooks devoted twice the space to sweet cakes, cookies, and pastries as their British counterparts. Thus, the temptations and norms in each country, much like modern times, were uniquely their own.

How did Americans view themselves? It was in the late 1800s that gluttony became synonymous with fatness. And by the early 1900s, society had firmly turned against its obese members. At this time, synonyms for overweight emerged: porky, tubby, sod-packer, jumbo, and butterball (Schwartz 1986, 89).

The late 1800s also saw a trimming down of formal dinners in number of courses and length. Yet they were not economical affairs. Take the life insurance medical directors dinner from 1895, where the menu was clams, cream soup, kingfish, new potatoes, filet mignon, string beans, sweetbreads, green peas, squab, asparagus, petits fours, cheese, coffee, and liqueurs (Schwartz 1986, 91)!

Americans really began to know their own obesity at this time because of another innovation—the home scale. Over the course of the second half of the 19th century, the size of scales progressively decreased, and in 1891 the Fairbanks Scale Company designed scales portable enough for use in hotels, clubs, and athletic facilities. They could also be found in doctors' offices, insurance examiners' offices, grocery stores, and drug stores. The scales designed to measure the weight of a man or woman were called "penny scales" and included a chart documenting ideal weight for height and a mirror. Penny scales were enormously popular and could also be found in train stations, restaurants, five-and-dime stores, and the lobbies of movie theaters, banks, and office buildings. There was even one in Chicago's City Hall in 1922. In 1927, the penny scale industry was a $5 million business.

Around this time, more and more Americans had indoor private bathrooms (half the country by 1930), and with this came an interest in personal scales for the bathroom that were smaller and, more important, more private, than penny scales or those in doctors' offices. The first patent on a bathroom scale was issued in 1916 to Mathias Weber. Mathias teamed up with two investors and began selling the Health-O-Meter bathroom scale in 1919.

Obesity invaded the home in other ways. The turn of the century also saw the rise of home economics and with it the rise of women writing about the dangers of obesity. It was now the housewife's job to monitor her own weight and the weight of her family, relying on domestic economy to avoid overabundance in consumption and weight.

It was also the time of ideal weights. Life insurance companies began examining the data of their policy holders, and in 1901 New York Life Insurance reported an analysis by Dr. Oscar Rogers of 1,553 men who were at least 30 percent overweight. These men had 34.5 percent higher mortality than men who were of average weight. Metropolitan Life company proclaimed, "The longer the belt line, the shorter the lifeline" (Schwartz 1986, 159). Based on a larger analysis of over 700,000 insured men, the insurance companies subsequently reported that being overweight was more dangerous than being underweight. Weight charts began shifting from the "average" weight to an "ideal" weight. Society responded by narrowing the range of perceived acceptable weights.

Advertisers picked up on the drive for smaller weights and responded in kind. Cigarette companies began pushing their product as a weight control in the late 1920s with taglines like "Reach for a Lucky instead of a sweet" (Schwartz 1986, 181).

Retail also responded to the increasing attention to body size. Ready-made clothing was coming into fashion, but sizings were based on Civil War measurements and Americans had grown much taller. Clothing styles were also losing their bulk and, with it, some of the weight-hiding ability of a full skirt. All of this made the times ripe for the arrival of Lena Bryant. Just before World War I, Lena's company, Lane Bryant (named because of a typing error by a clerk), began manufacturing clothing for larger women. Bryant got her start making maternity wear for working and middle-class women; in fact, she's believed to have made the first commercially available maternity dress. But her clothes for larger women quickly became the meat of the business, and the company continues to sell to that demographic to this day.

OBESITY IN MEDICINE

Modern scientific medicine began to emerge around the turn of the 16th century. Physicians started to conduct research into obesity. Nicholas Bonetus performed the first anatomical dissection of an obese person. In 1614, Santorio Santorio, considered the father of metabolic obesity, created a metabolic balance (see Figure 1.2). By standing on this and using counterweights, Santorio was able to measure the effect that food intake and excretion had on body weight. In the late 18th century, Lazzaro Spallanzani demonstrated that gastric liquid digested food.

Alexis St. Martin was a young French Canadian fur trapper working in the northern Michigan territory. In 1822, while working as a voyageur for the American Fur Company, he was accidentally shot by a musket. The shot, containing gunpowder and duck shot (small metal pellets), hit St. Martin in the abdomen, "literally blowing off integuments and muscles the size of a man's hand, fracturing and carrying away the anterior half of the sixth rib, fracturing the fifth, lacerating the lower portion of the left lobe of the lungs, the

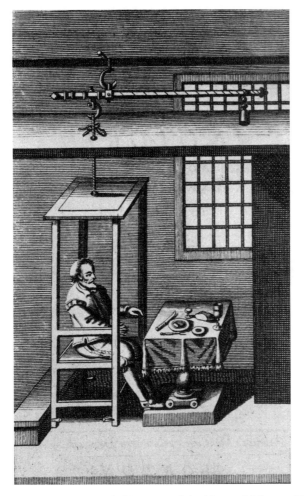

Figure 1.2. Santorio Santorio's scale [Courtesy of the National Library of Medicine].

diaphragm, and perforating the stomach," according to the physician, Dr. William Beaumont, who ultimately treated St. Martin. (Beaumont 1838, 8). Miraculously, St. Martin survived the incident and remained under Dr. Beaumont's care. In May 1925, Dr. Beaumont began taking advantage of the unique circumstances that Mr. St. Martin offered. The wound left a hole in St. Martin's side that allowed Beaumont to directly observe the stomach and its contents. As Beaumont continued treating St. Martin in the subsequent days, weeks, and years, he found the open hole in St. Martin's stomach allowed all that he consumed to pass out of the digestive system. It also allowed Beaumont to directly observe the digestive process. His observations, published in 1838, provided physicians with a wealth of information about how the digestive system works.

Beaumont's medical work had important implications in society at large, which at the time was struggling with the notion of hunger. Many believed hunger was a moral and spiritual choice. But Beaumont's work with Alexis St. Martin was suggesting hunger was a physiologic phenomenon residing in the stomach. Did the head listen to the stomach or the stomach to the head? It is a notion that continues to pervade dietary advice to this day as some diets emphasize the notion of letting the stomach dictate when you eat and others provide all number of tricks to "fool" the stomach into eating less or later.

Working in Germany in the middle of the 19th century, Justus von Liebig identified that humans need carbohydrates, protein, and fat. His work provided the basis of nutritional science until the discovery of vitamins. Research on vitamins dominated much of nutritional science research in the first half of the 20th century. In 1879, George Hoggon and his wife, Dr. Francis Elizabeth Hoggon, outlined the growth and development of fat cells. In the 20th century, the works of several scientists led to the conclusion that hunger was correlated with stomach contractions. The first human calorimeter was constructed in 1896 at Wesleyan University in Connecticut. The inventors, Wilbur Olin Atwater and E. B. Rosa, used the device to study the metabolic requirements of humans during starvation and food intake. In the era we think of as modern medicine (dating after World War II), scientists continued to refine the calorimeter and used their findings to refine theories of obesity that included discussions of the metabolic rate, carbohydrate oxidation, and insulin sensitivity.

The end of the 1800s also saw the rise of a different kind of response to obesity—the hunger artist. These individuals starved themselves on the public stage and raised questions for medicine about what the minimum dietary requirements were. The most famous hunger artist of the time was Dr. Henry Tanner, who fasted for 40 days. After the first day, Tanner went without water for 14 days, at which point he relented and took in only water until the end of his fast. Tanner's fast was covered by newspapers around the world, and visitors paid 25 cents each to see Tanner during his fast. Around this time, fasting taken to an extreme, anorexia, was recognized as its own medical diagnosis.

Early in the 20th century, Archibald Garrod defined metabolic disorders, thus beginning our associations of obesity with metabolism. In 1923, Charles Davenport noted how high body size ran in families, beginning the discussion of the heritability of obesity. The year 1992 marked another milestone in the genetics of obesity, with the identification of a gene that caused obesity in mice. We'll talk more about the genetics of obesity in later chapters.

Throughout history, physicians, scientists, and skilled businessmen have offered pharmacologic therapies for obesity that include hydrotherapy (water treatment), laxatives, thyroid extract, testicular gland extract, aniline, and amphetamines. Nearly all have had disastrous side effects. For example, the most common aniline, dinitrophenol, was introduced as a weight-loss treatment after significant weight loss was seen in workers who handled the chemical. It was abandoned when high rates of cataracts and neuropathy were found in those who took it. We'll take a look at modern obesity drugs in Chapter 5.

Obesity treatments have a long history of their own. Hippocrates suggested "hard work" before food in the 5th century BCE. Galen suggested running. The 18th century brought about more medicalized treatments that included bleeding and purging in addition to exercise and a restricted diet. Advocating for a restrictive diet and exercise, perhaps the most common modern diet advice, is not new.

The early 1800s saw the rise of health reformer Sylvester Graham, who despite all his efforts will forever be known most as the inventor of the graham cracker. Graham became a minister after a childhood of ill health, serving as a guest minister and then as a temperance lecturer. He saw, as did many Christians of the time, stimulation as bad for the body and soul. As a temperance lecturer, Graham preached of the ills of alcohol as a stimulant, and this segued nicely into his role as a health reformer, in which he decried the inflammatory effects not just of alcohol but also of all beverages aside from water as well as spices, condiments, meat, and a sedentary life. Graham also spoke of the risks of eating things not "natural," like white flour (which resulted when the wheat and bran were separated in processing). Interestingly, in modern times, health reformers also caution against inflammation and consumption of overprocessed foods like white bread. While the reasons for Graham's message were quite different from the reasons we'll talk about in this book, parts of his message are apparent in modern health messages. Followers of Graham, and his contemporary William Alcott, were often gaunt and pale. Many "Grahamites," as they were known, came to the health movement as a last resort for existing illnesses. That didn't stop many in society from mocking the movement. Grahamites created the nation's first health food store, supplying whole-wheat (Graham) bread and fresh fruits and vegetables (grown in unadulterated soil). They also created houses where they could live with fellow Grahamites and published journals that emphasized the benefits of their lifestyle. Grahamites and those who scoffed at their lifestyle looked at each other with mutual disdain. Alcott penned a prayer about the lifestyle of the populace, which begins

Give us this day our daily bread
And pies and cakes besides
To load the stomach, pain the head
And choke the vital tides.
And if too soon a friend decays,
Or dies in agony—
We'll talk of God's mysterious ways
And lay it all to thee.

(Whorton 1982, 54)

In contrast, skeptics of the Graham way of life speculated that dinner at a Graham house was a sad site with residents gathered around groaning at "straggling radishes, ... a soggy bunch of asparagus, ... corpses of potatoes, ... a thin segment of bran bread, and a tumbler of cold water" (Whorton 1982, 59). The Graham way of life was far reaching. Oberlin College, the first coeducational college in the nation and the first to admit black students on an equal basis with white students, instituted Grahamism, eliminating meat from the dining table at the school. The campus community soon revolted (town residents even suspected the students were being starved), and the president of the college, an ardent Grahamite, was dismissed.

Graham's story is not unique. In fact, fitness and obesity historian James Whorton noted that many of the health reformers have followed a standard biography:

Weak constitution or bad habits
Descent through levels of vitality to semi invalidism
Shock at poor health leads to renunciation of the existing lifestyle and search for an answer
Reading or self experimentation reveal the practice that is required for rebuilding health
Well being follows reform
Convincing the person that this is the secret
Giving him energy to compose articles/books which preach his message.

(Whorton 1982, 9)

While Whorton writes of this in describing the health reformer history of the mid-1800s to early 1900s, the story is a familiar one and may remind us of more modern advocates of fad diets who advocate them after a personal success. Increasingly, these advocates often take to disparaging the science supporting alternative approaches and ignore the data questioning the efficacy of their preferred approach.

Later, in 1826, Jean Anthelme Brillat-Savarin suggested discretion in eating, moderation in sleeping, and exercise to battle the bulge. The first popular diet book arrived in 1863, by William Banting. It was actually a pamphlet titled *Letter on Corpulence, Addressed to the Public* and contained the details of the low-carbohydrate diet that led to Banting's own weight loss. Banting described the diet he had been following and the one he adopted, which he believed was the key to his subsequent 50-pound weight loss. The diet he had followed included "bread, butter, milk, sugar, beer, and potatoes." Banting described his new diet as the following general plan:

For breakfast, I take five to six ounces of beef, mutton, kidneys, broiled fish, bacon, or cold meat of any kind except pork; a large cup of tea (without milk or sugar), a little biscuit, or one ounce of dry toast.

For dinner, Five or six ounces of any fish except salmon, any meat except pork, any vegetable except potato, one ounce of dry toast, fruit out of a pudding, any kind of poultry or game, and two or three glasses of good claret, sherry, or Madeira—Champagne, port, and beer forbidden.

For tea, Two or three ounces of fruit, a rusk or two, and a cup of tea without milk or sugar.

For supper, Three or four ounces of meat or fish, similar to dinner, with a glass or two of claret.

For nightcap, if required, A tumbler of grog—(gin, whisky, or brandy, without sugar)—or a glass or two of claret or sherry. (Banting 1863, 10)

Banting estimated that he consumed five or six ounces of solid food and eight ounces of liquid food at breakfast (typically eaten at 9:00 A.M. in Banting's time), eight ounces solid and eight of liquid at dinner (typically at 2:00 P.M.), three ounces of solid and eight of liquid at tea (typically at 6:00 P.M.), and four ounces solid and six of liquid at supper (typically at 9:00 P.M.).

Banting advocated lean meat, and the popularity of his method paved the way for the creation of the (in)famous Salisbury steak, a modern staple of school cafeterias and TV dinners. Dr. James Salisbury spent his career searching for the nutrition plan that would lead to health. He undertook study after study of diets of single foods in search of the answer and found many foods left "glue"-like remnants in the body, including meat. As a result, he advocated the consumption of hot water and the "muscle pulp of lean beef made into cakes and broiled" (Schwartz 1986, 102). Thus was born the Salisbury steak. Unfortunately for Dr. Salisbury, modern versions of the steak that bears his name are hardly seen as health food!

Other similar diets soon followed Banting's, including Van Noorden's low-fat, high-protein, high-carbohydrate diet and Ebstein's high-fat, low-carbohydrate diet. The basis for popular modern diets like Atkins and South Beach can be seen in these early works.

Later in the century brought the arrival of Horace Fletcher and his cure-all for obesity, which became known as Fletcherism. Fletcher was another who had a health crisis and was left overweight and searching for a cure in hygiene books. He came upon the notion that careful mastication (chewing) was necessary. At the time, Americans were widely derided for their eating habits. Europeans perceived Americans as sedentary and, more important, appalling eaters in quality, quantity, and speed. One typical portrait showed an American in front of a mountain of meat and starch, fried or loaded with butter. Interestingly, this isn't entirely different from the modern picture foreigners have of the American dining experience with our supersized meals and dining-on-the-run culture.

Fletcher became committed to slow eating through extensive chewing (100 chews per minute). Fletcher believed this approach would work as it was grounded in nature, and nature could not be wrong. Since the digestion of food was beyond his control, it was the work of nature, so the errors must be in the ingestion of food. Thus, he advocated eating only when hungry, choosing only the foods that were appealing at that moment, and eating only as long as one remained hungry. But the piece of advice Fletcher became most known for was that one should keep food in the mouth as long as the taste remained as taste was nature's gift of pleasure. By systematically chewing until all taste was gone from his food, Fletcher dropped from 205 pounds in January 1898 to 163 pounds in October. Fletcherism was enormously popular and was championed by many, including oil magnate John D. Rockefeller.

Fletcher also began asserting that the protein intakes of Americans were much too high. Fletcher claimed his superb physical fitness was due to his avoidance of excessive "indigestible" food, by which he meant too much protein in the diet. In fact, his fitness was confirmed through evaluation at the Yale University gym, where he consistently outperformed the university's varsity athletes despite his lack of physical training.

This, in part, led to evaluations by Dr. Russell Chittenden of how much protein was necessary. Fletcher's fame caught the attention of Dr. Chittenden, who invited Fletcher to Yale in 1902 to determine the smallest amount of food necessary to keep the body at maximum efficiency. At the time, conventional wisdom held that anywhere from 118 to 165 grams of protein per day were necessary. Yet Fletcher claimed to subsist on just 45 grams per day. Interestingly, the wisdom at the time was a function of the scientific focus on wealthy individuals and highlights a theme we'll return to later—namely, that findings found in wealthy individuals may not apply to other segments of the population or may provide a skewed perspective. The conclusion that at least 118 grams of protein were necessary came by analyzing the diets of wealthy individuals who could afford to eat as much as they wanted. It was premised on the (false) notion that the body would constrain people to eat only what they needed. Around the time of Chittenden's research on Fletcher's protein intake, other researchers in Europe were suggesting that as little as 15 grams per day might be sufficient. Not only did Chittenden's research suggest that much less protein was necessary than previously thought, but also some of his studies suggested that such high levels might actually be detrimental. He studied athletes and found that not only did their health not decline on the lower protein diets but their strength actually rose. Fletcher and Chittenden continued to work together through 1906.

Fletcher also influenced Yale economist Irving Fisher to examine whether Fletcherizing improved endurance, which might increase the productivity of the U.S. worker. Fisher's experiment found students who followed Fletcher's plan of thorough mastication, obedience to appetite, and reduced protein intake saw improvements in endurance.

In the early 1900s Americans also began a new approach to the battle of the bulge—calorie counting. The focus wasn't on addition (total intake) but on trade-offs: If I walk *this* long, it will offset the calories in a cookie. Viennese physician Gustav Gaertner wrote *Reducing Weight Comfortably*, which advocated a low-calorie, high-anxiety diet. Dr. Lulu Hunt Peters wrote the first bestselling diet book, *Diet and Health with Key to the Calories*, in 1918. The first page of Peters' book provided a simple formula for calculating ideal weight:

Multiply number of inches over 5 feet by $5\frac{1}{2}$ and add 110.
    So 5 feet 5 inches without shoes would be:
    $5 \times 5.5 = 27.5 + 110 = 137.5$ pounds

Though this was not the first formula of its kind, Peters' program provided an integration of the previous 50 years of obesity science. Her program begins with a fast and follows with a low-calorie diet and Fletcherizing. Peters worked in 100-calorie portions and advocated the lower protein portions suggested by Chittenden and Fletcher's work at Yale. Peters' plan was for lifelong calorie counting.

The appeal of calorie counting at the turn of the century was limited because science did not yet understand differences in metabolism between individuals. Thus, two people consuming the same number of calories could have wildly different responses. Struggling to understand the different responses of obese individuals to intervention, two kinds of obesity were described in the medical literature: endogenous and exogenous (see Table 1.1). Exogenous obesity resulted from a misguided appetite and resulted in too many calories taken in. Endogenous obesity was the result of an unhealthy metabolism and not enough calories being burned.

Exogenous obesity could be treated by a lean diet, but endogenous obesity was less responsive and required something else. That something turned out to be thyroid extract. Thyroid extract was first given as an obesity treatment in 1893. In 1896, iodine was shown to be a significant component of thyroid

Table 1.1
The Two Kinds of Obesity in 1900

	Exogenous	Endogenous
Other names	Sthenic	Asthenic
	Plethoric	Anemic
	Alimentary	Constitutional
Seen most in	Men	Women
Due to	Overeating	Deficient metabolism
Location of fat	Stomach	Abdomen, breasts, hips
Distribution	Symmetrical	Asymmetrical
Texture	Solid	Flabby
General health	Good	Poor
Disposition	Cheerful	Sad or sour
Appearance	Ruddy	Pale, bloated
Appetite	Keen	Capricious
Skin	Soft, smooth	Wrinkled, pimpled
Muscles	Firm	Flaccid (atonic)
Heart	Vigorous	Feeble
Blood	Full, rich	Thin, poor
Blood pressure	High	Low
Temperature	Normal	Abnormal
Pathologies	Heart problems	Diabetes
Remedies	Reduced diet	Electrotherapy
	Exercise	Massage
	Laxatives	Thyroid drugs
Prognosis	Good when young	Poor at all times

Source: Schwartz (1986, 137).

hormone. Iodine had been used as a treatment for obesity since the mid-1800s and was the key ingredient in one of the most popular medications for obesity of the time—Allan's Anti-Fat. By 1910, the market was flooded with iodine-containing fat treatments. They were enormously popular despite warnings of significant side effects, including tachycardia. To offset these heart-related side effects, many doctors prescribed a drug cocktail of thyroid extract mixed with arsenic or strychnine. Other doctors insisted on strict monitoring of patients on iodine because of the potential complications. Thus began a real medicalization of obesity.

Calorie counting returned to prominence at the start of World War I when concerns over food shortages (especially of fat and sugar) were front and center. Ad campaigns spoke of the "gospel of the clean plate" and described U-boats and wastefulness as twin enemies. Being fat was now unpatriotic as it suggested consuming more than one's share in a time of shortages.

Dr. Luella Axtell was the first woman to open an obesity clinic around this time. Dr. Axtell was skeptical of drugs and diets and instead advocated exercise, massage, and short-term, low-calorie diets.

The end of the 1800s also gave rise to obesity treatment centers. John Harvey Kellogg was head of the Seventh-day Adventist sanitarium in Battle Creek, Michigan, the chief hydrotherapy center in the United States at the time (see Figure 1.3). Battle Creek's list of obesity treatments included a cold rain douche, sweating packs, cold dripping sheets, short plunge baths, electric arc light baths, and sun baths. Guests at the sanitarium over time included many famous Americans such as John D. Rockefeller, J. C. Penney, Montgomery Ward, Myrtle Walgreen, and S. S. Kresge, the founder of Kmart. By 1935, 300,000 people had visited Battle Creek and millions more had read Kellogg's writings.

Kellogg's fame came in part from his multipronged approach to obesity treatment. An admirer of Graham, in 1877 Kellogg created a breakfast cereal that followed Graham's approach to grains and was based on the formula of another of Graham's followers. Kellogg baked several grains and water into a hard biscuit, which he then ground and baked twice more. He called this granola. But Kellogg wasn't satisfied with the product and reworked it again, tempering it into flakes in 1893. Kellogg's brother Will added malt and sugar to John Harvey's corn flake, and by 1929 Will Kellogg had sold 50 million packages of his corn flakes despite over 100 other brands of corn flake being made in Battle Creek because of Will Kellogg's failure to patent his recipe. John Harvey felt the digestive system needed purification and worked with his brother to create a bran cereal that would aid that process. Kellogg's All-Bran cereal became a key part of a weight-reducing diet by providing bulk and iron.

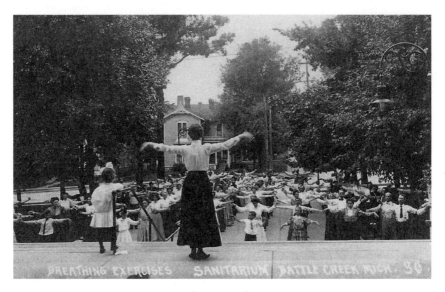

Figure 1.3. Battle Creek Sanitarium [Wikipedia].

John Harvey Kellogg also created a passive exercise machine that used an oscillating current and stocked the Battle Creek Sanitarium with vibrating chairs and machines to beat and massage fat away.

The 20th century saw the rise of behavior modification efforts in obesity treatment, beginning with Richard B. Stuart, who advocated that successful weight loss occurred when the environment for eating was changed and intake monitored. Thinking began to shift from biology to psychology as clinicians asked *why* we ate so much. Many theories conveniently blamed mothers—either for abandoning their children to the workforce or for smothering them! Groups focused on weight loss began forming in the late 1940s, with TOPS (Take Off Pounds Sensibly) followed in the 1960s by Overeaters Anonymous, Weight Watchers, and Diet Workshop.

While we think of fad diets as being something new, a review of the history of obesity diets suggests the only thing that changes are the names and the secret ingredient du jour. And many of the remedies introduced in the late 1800s and early 1900s were not new at all but regurgitations of age-old fat busters and treatments: vinegars, lotions, salts, soaps, and drinks. Citric acid was a common component of popular remedies like Russell's Anti-Corpulent Preparation, Every Woman's Flesh Reducer, and Jean Down's Get Slim. The same medicines that were used previously to treat indigestion were repackaged as fat dissolvers like Densmore's Corpulence Cure. But this era also saw the introduction of some truly new obesity treatments, including Fletcherism, fasting, and calorie counting. It was also the beginning of an era when thyroid-insufficiency drugs were used to ramp up metabolism.

After the risks of thyroid medications came the rise in popularity of dinitrophenol, a benzene derivative in the 1930s. Those taking dinitrophenol lost two to three pounds more per week than those on laxatives or thyroid extract, but the side effects included feeling warm, perspiration, rash, loss of taste sensations, cataract-induced blindness, and death. People also began taking Benzedrine, an amphetamine. This approach was particularly popular with men. By the 1970s, 8 percent of all prescription medications were for amphetamines, and one-fourth of those were being used for weight loss.

While the 1800s had citric acid and vinegar, the modern explosion of diet fads includes the grapefruit diet, no high-fructose corn syrup diet, maple syrup diet, macrobiotic diet, cabbage soup diet, and Scarsdale diet. Alas, some of these are not so new. The Beverly Hills diet that gained popularity in the 1980s is simply the 1920s Medical Millennium diet of Dr. William Hay, who advocated consuming one food per meal. Starches were to be eaten separately from protein and both separately from fruit. Careful chewing (Fletcherizing arises again!) and colonic cleansing were also part of Hay's plan.

Some commercial diets are simply glorified versions of these fad diets while other commercial diets have actually undergone some scientific evaluation. Why do these fad diets that lack scientific evidence gain popularity and last in our memories? Many of the most popular follow a formula (intentional or not) of celebrity + weight loss = latest fad diet. Supplements have a similar history. One has only to look at the images of Anna Nicole Smith's weight loss and ubiquitous presence in weight-loss supplement ads for evidence. Yet there is almost no scientific evaluation of the merits of any of these supplements at achieving sustained weight loss, and many have adverse side effects.

Surgical treatment for obesity dates back to the third century. Early efforts sought to remove excess fat. The first modern lipectomy was in 1889 by Howard Kelly at Johns Hopkins, who cut layers of fat from abdomens of patients in the hospital for other surgeries. By the 1920s surgery was an accepted treatment for severe obesity. More modern approaches include bypassing parts of the digestive system, such as the jejunoileal bypass introduced by Kremen in 1954 and the gastric bypass introduced by Mason and Ito in 1970. We'll take a closer look at surgical treatment for obesity in Chapter 5.

As we look at the modern prevention and treatment approaches to obesity, we'll see parallels with historic approaches. Despite the wealth of modern data we'll review on the consequences of obesity, much of what is offered for obesity treatment isn't entirely new.

2

What Is Obesity?

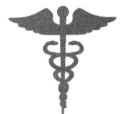

ADULTS

Obesity in adults is typically defined using body mass index (BMI), a measure of weight to height (see Figure 2.1). A BMI of 30 kilograms (kg) per meter squared (m^2) is considered obese, while a BMI between 25 and 29.9 is considered overweight. The use of weight divided by height squared as a measure of body fatness was first proposed in 1869 by Adolphe Quetelet and is thus also called Quetelet's Index. The purpose of weight for height indices is that they produce a measure of weight that is independent of height. For example, if we take two individuals, each weighing 180 lb., and ask if either is overweight, the answer is "it depends." If Joe is five feet, five inches tall and John is six feet, two inches tall, it is easy to imagine how different 180 lb at each height is. This is evident if we calculate a BMI for each: Joe's BMI is 30 and he would be considered obese, while John's BMI is 23.7 and he is considered normal weight.

In the United States, 66 percent of adults are overweight or obese and 32 percent of adults are obese, and these numbers show a trend of increasing over time. Of particular concern is the rapid increase in the prevalence of morbid obesity (BMI $\geq$ 40 kg/m^2) in young adults; in 1999 just 4.5 percent of U.S.

BMI	19	20	21	22	23	24	25	26	27	28	29	30	31	32	33	34	35	36	37	38	39	40
Height inches											Body Weight pounds											
58	91	96	100	105	110	115	119	124	129	134	138	143	148	153	158	162	167	172	177	181	186	191
59	94	99	104	109	114	119	124	128	133	138	143	148	153	158	163	168	173	178	183	188	193	198
60	97	102	107	112	118	123	128	133	138	143	148	153	158	163	168	174	179	184	189	194	199	204
61	100	106	111	116	122	127	132	137	143	148	153	158	164	169	174	180	185	190	195	201	206	211
62	104	109	115	120	126	131	136	142	147	153	158	164	169	175	180	186	191	196	202	207	213	218
63	107	113	118	124	130	135	141	146	152	158	163	169	175	180	186	191	196	202	207	214	220	225
64	110	116	122	128	134	140	145	151	157	163	169	174	180	186	191	197	203	208	214	221	227	232
65	114	120	126	132	138	144	150	156	162	168	174	180	186	192	197	204	209	215	221	228	234	240
66	118	124	130	136	142	148	155	161	167	173	179	186	192	198	204	210	216	222	228	235	241	247
67	121	127	134	140	146	153	159	166	172	178	185	191	198	204	210	216	223	229	235	242	249	255
68	125	131	138	144	151	158	164	171	177	184	190	197	204	210	217	223	230	236	242	249	256	262
69	128	135	142	149	155	162	169	176	182	189	196	203	210	216	223	230	236	243	249	257	263	270
70	132	139	146	153	160	167	174	181	188	195	202	209	216	222	230	236	243	250	257	264	271	278
71	136	143	150	157	165	172	179	186	193	200	208	215	222	229	236	243	250	257	265	272	279	286
72	140	147	154	162	169	177	184	191	199	206	213	221	228	235	242	250	258	265	272	279	287	294
73	144	151	159	166	174	182	189	197	204	212	219	227	235	242	250	257	265	272	280	288	295	302
74	148	155	163	171	179	186	194	202	210	218	225	233	241	249	256	264	272	280	287	295	303	311
75	152	160	168	176	184	192	200	208	216	224	232	240	248	256	264	272	279	287	295	303	311	319
76	156	164	172	180	189	197	205	213	221	230	238	246	254	263	271	279	287	295	304	312	320	328

Figure 2.1. Body mass index [Courtesy of National Institute of Diabetes and Kidney Diseases. Redrawn by Jeff Dixon.].

adults were in the extreme obesity category, but this rose to 5.4 percent in just four years. The maps in Figure 2.2 show how the prevalence of obesity has increased in the United States over the last 30 years. A year-by-year version of the maps can be found at http://www.cdc.gov/nccdphp/dnpa/obesity/trend/maps. As the prevalence of obesity in a state increases, the color of the state gets darker, and by 1997, a new color had to be introduced to account for the rising rates of obesity. While the rates of obesity have been increasing steadily from the 1960s, rates of overweight are actually quite consistent. In 1960, the prevalence of overweight was 31.5 percent and the prevalence of obesity was 13.3 percent. By 2001, the prevalence of overweight was 33.9 percent but the prevalence of obesity had risen to 32.1 percent.

Percentage of U.S. Adults with BMI > 30, or 30 lb. overweight for 5'4" person

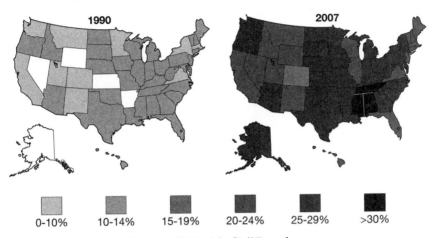

Figure 2.2. Obesity trends among U.S. adults [Jeff Dixon].

These data are based on self-report of height and weight. This is a concern because we know that people like to see themselves in the best light, and as a result they tend to think of themselves as taller and thinner than they really are. Consequently, the prevalence of obesity in the United States is likely even greater than we think.

Also troubling is the fact that obesity rates are not equivalent across groups. Minorities, the poor, and women are all more likely to be obese. In 2003, 45 percent of non-Hispanic blacks and 36.8 percent of Mexican Americans were obese as compared to 30.6 percent of non-Hispanic whites. Also, 33 percent of women as compared to 31 percent of men were obese, but within those groups, racial and ethnic disparities exist. For example, 54 percent of black women are obese as compared to 34 percent of black men, 30 percent of white women, and 31 percent of white men. The prevalence of overweight and obesity combined is also markedly higher among African Americans and Hispanics. Currently, there is about a 14 to 21 percentage point difference in the prevalence of overweight and obesity among non-Hispanic black (78 percent), Mexican American (71.8 percent), and white women (57.5 percent). The difference in the prevalence of overweight and obesity varies by approximately 8 to 14 percentage points among non-Hispanic black (60.1 percent), Mexican American (74.4 percent), and white men (67.5 percent) (Y. Wang and Bedoun 2008). Asian Americans have the lowest prevalence of obesity. The prevalence of overweight and obesity among Asian American adults is lower (33 percent) as compared to other ethnic/racial groups (Y. Wang et al. 2007).

African Americans and Hispanics are the largest minority groups in the United States, and the Hispanic population is growing rapidly. Studies tend to include information about these groups, but information is not as abundant for Asian populations. National studies may not accurately estimate the prevalence of obesity among certain ethnic and racial groups, such as Hawaiians or Pacific Islanders, because too few are included in the sample. As a result, we do not have a full picture of the prevalence of obesity in some minority groups.

It is also important to note that there is a lot of diversity within racial and ethnic groups. Asking someone to identify their race or ethnicity based on just a few categories lumps together people who may be from a wide geographic area with many different cultural behaviors and food traditions. For example, when people identify themselves as Asian American, they could be Vietnamese American, Chinese American, Japanese American, Thai American, Indian American, or many other nationalities. Yet it is important to measure overweight and obesity among different racial and ethnic groups because it gives researchers and health workers a bird's-eye view of the extent of the problem, even if the estimate is not precise. In addition, some surveys allow respondents to select only one racial or ethnic category, which is problematic in an increasingly multiethnic population like the United States.

Finally, the higher prevalence rates of overweight and obesity among the different ethnic and racial minority groups have the potential to increase the disease burden among these populations.

CHILDREN

In children, a weight-for-height index is also used, but the cutoff points for identifying those whose body fat puts them at increased risk of disease are different. Instead of using an absolute cutoff point as in adults, in children and adolescents relative cutoff points based on percentiles for age and gender are used. Beginning in 1998, children whose BMIs were between the 85th and 95th percentiles were considered at risk of overweight, and those in the 95th percentile or above were considered overweight. In 2007, an expert panel recommended changing the terminology to define those at or above the 95th percentile as obese and children between the 85th and 95th percentiles as overweight. The aim of the terminology change was to more accurately reflect the significant increased risk of adverse health outcomes in children at or above the 95th percentile and to reduce confusion about the "at risk of overweight" term. As has been the case throughout, these cutoff points do not apply to children under age two. To be consistent, we will use the 2007 recommended terms throughout this text.

Adiposity in children changes with age, which is why percentiles are always age specific. BMI in children increases until between eight months and 1 year of age and then declines until the child is between 4 and 7 years, when it increases again. When a child reaches the nadir of his or her BMI at a younger age, the risk of overweight as an adolescent or adult is increased. The number of fat cells (adipocytes) in children increases after age 10, but the size of the fat cells is typically stable from late infancy to adolescence. In overweight children, the fat cells increase to their adult size in infancy and stay that way through adolescence.

In 2003 in the United States, 33.6 percent of children and adolescents were overweight or obese; 17 percent of children and adolescents were obese. The increasing prevalence of obesity is alarming; in 1999 just 14 percent of children and adolescents were obese. As with adults, the prevalence of obesity in Mexican American and non-Hispanic black children and adolescents is significantly higher than among non-Hispanic whites.

According to national estimates, the prevalence of obesity among children and adolescents has tripled since 1980. The prevalence of overweight is greater among African American and Hispanic children and adolescents, with the exception of adolescent boys. Among 6- to 11-year-old children, non-Hispanic black girls (26.5 percent) and Mexican American boys (25.3 percent) have the highest prevalence of overweight. The prevalence of overweight among white girls and boys was 16.9 percent and 18.5 percent, respectively. Among adolescents (ages 12 to 19), the prevalence of overweight was highest among non-Hispanic black girls (25.4 percent). The prevalence of overweight among adolescent boys was between 18 and 19 percent for all ethnicities. The prevalence among white adolescent girls and boys was 15.4 percent. The prevalence of obesity (BMI $\geq$ 30) among Native American children is 39 percent for boys and 14 percent for girls (Y. Wang 2007).

Analysis of data from the 2003–2004 National Survey of Children's Health estimated that a higher proportion of African American (49.2 percent) and Hispanic children (44.0 percent) were overweight as compared to Caucasian children (32.2 percent) (Lutfiyya et al. 2008).

A study of racial and ethnic differences in overweight and obesity among three-year-old children found that Hispanic children were two times more likely to be overweight or obese than either white or black children. In addition, a child's likelihood of being obese is higher if his or her mother is obese. The proportion of obese or overweight three-year-olds who had an obese mother was 42 percent for white, 36 percent for black, and 56 percent for Hispanic kids. In comparison, the proportion of obese or overweight three-year-olds who had mothers who were of normal weight was 26 percent for whites, 25 percent for blacks, and 40 percent for Hispanics (Kimbro et al. 2007).

A recently published study used U.S. national data on obesity from the last 30 years to calculate the proportion of people in the population who would be overweight or obese in the future. If current obesity trends continue, it is estimated that by 2030 51.1 percent of adults will be obese, 86.3 percent will be overweight or obese, 29.7 percent of children ages 6 to 11 years will be overweight, and 31 percent of adolescents ages 12 to 19 years will be overweight. By 2030, 96.9 percent of black women and 91.1 percent of Mexican American men will be overweight or obese. These groups are expected to have the highest proportions of overweight and obesity. The study projects that if trends continue, by 2048 *all* Americans age 20 and older will be categorized as overweight or obese (Y. Wang et al. 2008)! Some caution against such extrapolation as it assumes all trends are linear, which may not be the case. For example, if we extrapolate other data, then marathoners may have negative times some day in the future (Bialik 2008).

MEASUREMENT AND DIAGNOSIS

Adults

As we mentioned previously, BMI is the most commonly used measure of obesity. This is because BMI is easy (and cheap!) to measure. But BMI can be a poor proxy for body fatness in some groups—the elderly and particularly elite athletes. One certainly doesn't think of elite NFL running backs like LaDainian Tomlinson as being obese, but at five feet, 10 inches and 220 pounds, his BMI clocks in at 31.7, solidly in the obese range. The reason we don't think of "LT" as obese is that we know he packs a lot of muscle onto that five-foot, 10-inch frame. Similarly, a study of NBA players found half would be considered overweight based on their BMIs (Ritter 2005). BMI also doesn't tell us where the fat is located or what percentage of body weight is fat versus muscle. So what might be a better measure of fatness for athletes, or anyone else?

BMI is an indirect measure: We aren't directly measuring body fat but are using the weight-for-height index as a proxy. There are several ways of directly measuring body fatness. Underwater weighing measures body density. Since fat is less dense than water, the density of a person with more fat is lower. By weighing a person in air and under water, we can estimate the volume and percentage of body fat. This approach is the gold standard for determining body fatness, but it is time consuming and complicated. It is particularly challenging to measure the body fatness of children, the elderly, and the morbidly obese via underwater weighing. The facilities required for this are also limited. Can you imagine if every doctor's office had a big pool you had to get into at each visit instead of stepping on the scale?

Instead of measuring displaced water, air displacement instruments measure changes in air pressure. The most commonly used air displacement chamber is the Bod Pod (see Figure 2.3). This approach is easier with kids and the elderly, but it tends to underestimate body fat slightly.

Hydrometry estimates fat-free mass using dilution equations based on the body's excretion of ingested water that has been labeled with harmless radioactive isotopes. A carefully weighed dose of labeled water is consumed after fasting. A sample of blood or urine is typically collected before and about three to four hours after consuming the water. Body weight is calculated based on the dilution of the isotopes by total body fluid. It is a relatively easy procedure to

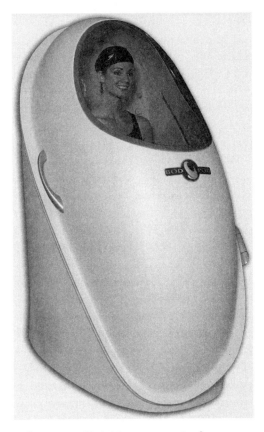

Figure 2.3. Bod Pod [Courtesy of Life Measurement, Inc.].

administer, but its accuracy depends on the precise measurement and dosing as well as accurate equations.

Body mass and fat can also be measured using imaging techniques like computed tomography (CT) scans and magnetic resonance imaging (MRI). These imaging techniques estimate body composition and fat distribution by taking scans of different cross sections of the body. They have advantages over other techniques in that they allow us to measure the amounts of different types of fat (visceral versus subcutaneous) and to measure the amount of fat around an organ or in a specific body region. They tend not to be used to estimate whole body fat as they are quite expensive and require special equipment that is not readily available.

A popular emerging technology is dual-energy x-ray absorptiometry (DXA). This scanning technique allows us to estimate fat mass as well as fat-free mass and bone mineral density. It is increasingly used in clinical practices, particularly among the elderly, to measure bone mass. It is simple, quick, and extremely precise but requires expensive equipment and can't be used on pregnant women or the morbidly obese. It is increasingly being considered the gold-standard approach for measuring body composition. However, unlike the technology provided by CT and MRI, DXA does not distinguish between visceral and subcutaneous fat.

Several indirect measures of body composition are also frequently used. Bioelectrical impedance analysis (BIA) passes an electrical current through the body. It operates under the premise that the current moves quicker through lean mass than fat mass and uses a prediction equation to estimate fat-free mass and percentage of body fat. The equations are population specific. BIA shows high correlations with estimates of the percentage of body fat derived from DXA and has the advantage that the equipment required is inexpensive, portable, and simple to use. However, some data suggest that BIA may not predict body fatness significantly better than BMI, which is cheaper and easier to measure.

What are the advantages and disadvantages of using BMI to measure body fatness? While several weight-for-height indices exist, BMI is the most frequently used because it has the highest correlation with adiposity as measured by densitometry. It is highly correlated with percentage of fat and total fat mass. BMI is easy and inexpensive to measure. While BMI can be calculated from self-reports of height and weight, its accuracy is correlated with the precision and accuracy of the height and weight measures, and we know that people tend to overestimate their height and underestimate their weight. BMI has other limitations, including the natural variations in the ratios of fat to lean mass that occur across age, sex, and racial or ethnic groups. At the same BMI, women have a greater percentage of body fat than men, and BMI is not gender specific.

As noted above, BMI is a proxy measure, and the most universally used, for body fatness. It is used because it correlates well with direct measures of body fat in most individuals. The exception is among the elderly, who tend to lose muscle mass as they age, and as such BMI may underestimate body fat.

Children

BMI is also the most commonly used measure of body fatness in children. The terminology for describing overweight in children is the subject of increasing debate. Those who advocate against using the term "obese" to describe children in the 95th percentile and above worry that the stigma associated with the term will have detrimental psychological effects. In addition, a child who appears overweight at one time point may subsequently achieve a BMI in the normal range. However, as noted previously, using different terms for children and adults has led to confusion, and the term "at risk of overweight" has confused some parents and practitioners, leading them to underestimate the health risks associated with a BMI between the 85th and 95th percentiles.

Body fatness can also be estimated by measuring skinfold thickness. Here, a set of calipers are used to pinch sections of skin and the subcutaneous fat. Prediction equations are used to estimate total body fat from the estimate of subcutaneous fat. Skinfold thickness measures have a high degree of variability between individuals taking the measurement and thus have a low reproducibility (the ability to get the same result at two separate measures). Skinfold thickness has limited value in the morbidly obese.

BODY FAT DISTRIBUTION

Up until this point, we have been talking mostly about measures of total body fat or percentage of body fat. However, research has suggested that the distribution of body fat may be as important as total body fat. In talking about the distribution of body fat, clinicians and researchers often consider pear and apple body shapes. Apple-shaped individuals carry most of their body fat around their abdomen while pear-shaped bodies carry the fat around the hips and thighs. Apple-shaped individuals are at a higher risk of diabetes, heart disease, and some cancers than pear-shaped individuals.

Waist-to-hip ratio and waist circumference are used to estimate the distribution of body fat. These are indirect measures of abdominal or central adiposity, which may be independently associated with risk of disease, separate from total body fatness. Waist circumference is strongly correlated with visceral fat. The challenge with these approaches is that because they are less frequently used we often see greater variability between measures. If you get on a scale three times, chances are that the weight the scale measures will be the same each time (if it isn't, you might want to get a new scale!). However, if you measure the waist circumference of your best friend three times, you are likely to get a slightly different answer each time as it requires practice and training to measure the exact same spot each time with the same amount of tension on the tape measure. Despite that, most people do reasonably well at measuring and reporting their waist circumference if given detailed instructions. As with BMI, interpretation of these indirect measures can be challenging as, for example, waist-to-hip ratio can be elevated because of a higher amount of fat mass or a lower amount of muscle mass.

In the elderly, measures of central adiposity, like waist circumference and waist-to-hip ratio, are better predictors of mortality than BMI because of the redistribution of fat as we age. Fat shifts from the arms and legs (peripheral areas) to the central torso area (abdomen) as we age. An elderly person's BMI may remain stable, but the fat has shifted location to the abdomen. Waist circumference and waist-to-hip ratio will both increase as a result of this, better reflecting the change in disease and mortality risk.

Want to know if you are an "apple" or a "pear"? If you are female and your waist-to-hip ratio is more than 0.8, you are an apple. If you are male and your waist-to-hip ratio is greater than 1.0, you are an apple. You can also just measure your waist. More than 40 inches for men or 35 for women indicates the high risk associated with central obesity or apple-shaped fat distributions.

Waist circumference has been shown to modify the risk of disease associated with BMI. If individuals have a high waist circumference (>40.2 inches in men, >34.6 inches in women) and are overweight, they are considered to be at high risk of cardiovascular disease (instead of just increased risk associated with being overweight). If individuals are obese with a high waist circumference, their risk of disease is very high. In the morbidly obese, risk of disease is extremely high regardless of waist circumference.

Knowing how obesity is measured and the extent of the problem provides a foundation for understanding the causes of obesity, the health risks associated with overweight and obesity, and the extent of efforts to prevent and treat it.

3

What Causes Obesity?

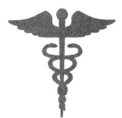

TIFFANY'S STORY

In the fall of 2008, a story in *The New York Times* profiled Tiffany King, a 12-year-old girl who at five feet tall weighed 354 pounds (Saul 2008). Tiffany wrote an essay that earned her a scholarship to a two-month weight-loss camp over the summer. There she managed to lose almost 40 pounds by the time a reporter interviewed her for the article a week before camp ended. The article highlighted the problem that there is little funding available to treat obese children. Tiffany was 1 of 173 kids to apply for only 10 spots at the camp in the summer of 2008. Most insurance plans do not cover the cost of weight-loss camps and selectively cover other treatments for obesity. And a lot of families cannot afford to send their children to camps that cost about $1,000 a week. In order to treat childhood obesity, doctors say it is important that treatment is available to many children throughout the year, not just in the summer. And a key component of treatment is to have parents involved. In addition, weight-loss camps may help kids lose weight, but it turns out that two-thirds of the kids gain the weight back. We'll talk about many of these issues Tiffany's story raises throughout this book.

At its simplest, obesity is caused by an energy imbalance—taking in more calories than one burns.

Caloric balance = energy in – energy out.
Energy out = basal metabolic rate + physical activity energy expenditure
+ thermic effect of food.

But other factors, like the environment, genetics, hormones, culture, and food choices, all contribute.

ENERGY IN

Energy in at the most basic level is the calories you consume, but in reality it is a complex interplay of many factors. Macronutrients (carbohydrates, protein, and fat), specific foods (or beverages), and eating patterns all play a role in the energy-in portion of the energy balance equation.

Fat is energy dense (more calories per gram) and makes foods more palatable. If we look at a macro level at fat intake across countries, we see that those countries consuming a greater percentage of calories from fat tend to have a higher prevalence of obesity (see Figure 3.1).

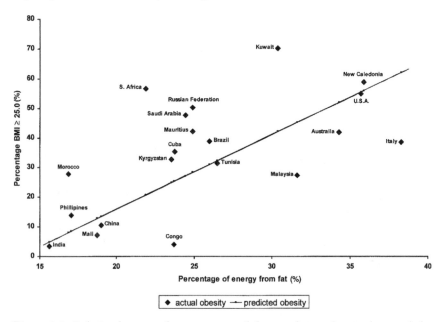

Figure 3.1. Relation between the percentage of the population that is obese and the proportion of energy intake from fat [Bray and Popkin 1998].

However, these countries differ on lots of other factors that also contribute to obesity, including level of economic development, food choices, and physical activity levels. In fact, if we adjust the fat intake for the level of economic development, the correlation mostly disappears. In studies that measure level of fat intake and follow a population forward in time, we see little evidence that a higher fat intake causes obesity. While some research has suggested that a decrease in the percentage of total calories from fat can result in weight loss, other data have indicated that the types of fats we eat might be most important, as high intakes of saturated and trans fats are associated with obesity.

Do carbohydrates cause obesity? There is some evidence that individuals who go on low-carbohydrate diets lose more weight in the short term than those on low-fat diets, but neither the difference nor the weight loss is sustained. Why might low-carbohydrate diets be more successful initially? Foods that are high in refined carbohydrates are thought to increase hunger and decrease feelings of satiety. As a result, individuals who consume diets high in refined carbohydrates often eat more calories overall. Thus, it isn't that carbohydrates directly cause excess weight gain but that they don't lead to feelings of satisfaction or fullness. Diets high in whole grains might help prevent weight gain because whole grains and unrefined carbohydrates also lead to feelings of satiety. In addition, these foods tend to be high in fiber and provide a low-calorie, bulky food that leaves one feeling full. Fruits and vegetables are low in calories and high in fiber and bulk, and diets high in both tend to be associated with lower rates of obesity.

The glycemic index (GI) is a tool that measures the effects that carbohydrates have on blood glucose levels. Carbohydrates that are easily and rapidly broken down lead to rapid releases of glucose into the blood and are considered high GI. Carbohydrates that break down slowly, leading to a gradual release of glucose into the blood, are low GI. Lower GI foods are thought to trigger slower digestion and absorption of sugar. Most fruits and vegetables, grainy breads, and legumes are low GI. Whole-wheat foods and brown rice are both medium GI, while white potatoes, white rice, and white bread are high-GI foods. An association between a high-GI diet and a high body mass index (BMI) has been seen, and this is believed to be because high-GI foods have low satiety.

Consuming diets high in protein may minimize weight gain because proteins increase satiety (foods high in protein are low GI because they are low in carbohydrate). Proteins also require more energy to digest than carbohydrates.

Specific foods might also contribute to weight gain. A growing body of research has shown that children who consume sugar-sweetened beverages are more likely to be overweight and obese. Children who cut sugar-sweetened beverages out of their diets typically lose weight. Foods and beverages high in sugar are also high GI. Alcohol can also contribute to weight gain as it is high in calories and can act as an appetite stimulant.

THE WAY WE EAT

Much has been made not only of what we eat but how and where we eat it. There is good evidence that eating breakfast helps prevent weight gain by moderating appetite-stimulating hormones. Certainly, the United States is eating out more. There is rapidly accumulating evidence that individuals who frequently eat at fast food restaurants are more likely to be overweight and obese. Fast food restaurants serve large portions of energy-dense food at a low price. This food is often highly palatable owing to the high fat content. But it is likely premature to say that these establishments *cause* obesity. If consumers didn't want the product offered, the businesses would fade away. Instead, fast food companies remain some of the most successful businesses in the United States, and Americans are eating out more than ever. Americans spent just 30 percent of their food budget on food eaten away from home in 1970, but by the late 1990s that figure had risen to nearly 50 percent. Perhaps it is simply that individuals who are already overweight or obese patronize these establishments. We also know that the foods most often served at fast food restaurants (high fat, high sugar, and energy dense) are strongly correlated with obesity.

We also know that portion sizes are increasing. Since the 1970s, portion sizes of most foods have increased significantly. In addition to increases in portions of food bought away from home, the portion sizes calculated for recipes for food cooked at home have increased.

When McDonald's introduced its french fries in 1955, there was one size and it was 2.4 oz. That size is now a McDonald's small, and the company offers a portion nearly three times that size (7.1 oz). McDonald's fries aren't alone—the same thing has happened across other fast food brands and for other fast food offerings like burgers and sodas. Coca-Cola's first offering in 1916 was a measly 6.5 oz., a size they don't even offer in 2008. Now the smallest can is 8 oz., and 34-oz. bottles are available. Hershey's first chocolate bar was 0.6 oz. in 1908, and today they offer sizes starting at 1.6 oz. and going up to 8 oz.— 13 times larger than the original (Young and Nestle 2003)!

Other evidence also suggests that the amount of food we are eating has increased over time. There has been a large increase in the availability of food in the United States, and while there has also been a corresponding increase in the amount of food that is wasted or thrown out, this doesn't entirely account for the increase in availability, suggesting that actual consumption has increased. However, most long-term studies that follow the same population over many years, recording what (and how much) individuals eat, find little evidence that the amount of food individuals consume has increased. Unfortunately, both types of studies suffer from errors in their measures of intake and waste, making it difficult to decide if one is more "right."

What Should We Eat? How Much?

The Harris-Benedict equation is a useful tool for adults to determine their caloric needs. It works like this. First, you need to calculate your basal metabolic rate (BMR). You can estimate this using the following formulas:

For women, BMR = 665 + (weight in pounds × 4.35) + (height in inches × 4.7) − (age in years × 4.7).
For men, BMR = 66 + (weight in pounds × 6.23) + (height in inches × 12.7) − (age in years × 6.8).

So the BMR for a 30-year-old woman who is five feet, 5 inches (65 inches) and 125 pounds is

665 + 543.75 + 305.5 − 141 = 1,373.25.

Then you need to account for your activity.

If you get little or no physical activity, your daily caloric need is BMR × 1.2.
If you get a little physical activity a few days a week (one to three days/ week), your daily caloric need is BMR × 1.375.
If you are moderately active, exercising three to five days/week, your daily caloric need is your BMR × 1.55.
If you are a heavy exerciser, exercising six or seven days/week, your daily caloric need is your BMR × 1.725.
Finally, if you are an extremely active person, exercising vigorously as with athletes in training, your daily caloric need is your BMR × 1.9.

So our 30-year-old woman, who exercises moderately, would need BMR × 1.55, or 1,373.25 × 1.55 = 2,128.5 calories per day
All of these figures are for the needs of someone looking to maintain his or her weight. To lose weight, one would need to consume less than this amount.

How Do We Get Those Calories?

The Food Guide Pyramid, developed by the U.S. Department of Agriculture (USDA), seeks to guide Americans about what they should eat and how

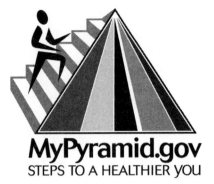

Figure 3.2. MyPyramid [USDA].

much of it they should eat (see Figure 3.2). In 2005, new guidelines were issued that advised the average person to eat the following:

- Grains: Eat 6 ounces every day.
- Vegetables: Eat 2.5 cups every day.
- Fruits: Eat 2 cups every day.
- Milk: Get 3 cups every day; for kids aged two to eight, it's 2 cups.
- Meat and beans: Eat 5.5 ounces every day.

Keep in mind that these are guidelines and that one set of recommendations does not fit all people. For example, women and children who are largely sedentary need less food. On the other hand, teenage boys who engage in a lot of physical activity will probably need more food.

The current recommendation for fruit and vegetable consumption is to eat 7 to 13 servings of fruits and vegetables a day. This recommendation is based on age, gender, and activity level. Many people find this recommendation daunting. In fact, a recent study showed that about 70 percent of Americans were not eating the amounts of fruits and vegetables recommended by the USDA (Thompson, O., unpublished data).

What's a Serving?

If you think that it is impossible to eat all the fruits and vegetables recommended each day, it is not as hard as you think. Think about 1 serving fitting in the palm of your hand! For example, a large salad is 2 to 4 servings of the vegetables you need per day, and eating a medium-sized apple means you have eaten half of the recommended 2.5 servings of fruit for one day (see Figure 3.3). When

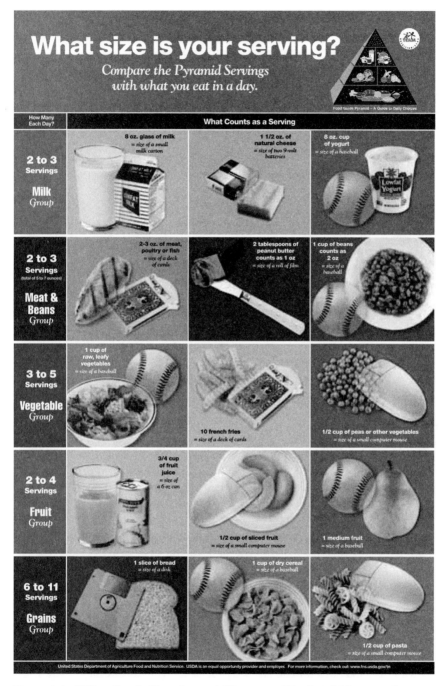

Figure 3.3. "What Size Is Your Serving? [Courtesy of Food and Nutrition Services, USDA].

you think about it, these serving sizes are a lot smaller than what we are used to seeing when we eat at restaurants or even at home.

Here are some examples of what counts as one serving:

- 0.5 cup of most fruits or vegetables
- 10 french fries
- 1 medium-sized piece of fruit, such as an apple
- 1 cup of raw leafy vegetables
- 0.5 cup of pasta, rice, or cereal
- 2–3 ounces of meat
- 0.5 cup of cooked beans
- 1 slice of bread
- 6 ounces of fruit or vegetable juice
- 8 ounces of milk

Unfortunately, most of us do a pretty bad job at estimating both serving sizes and how much we consume. In a Cornell University study, researchers offered moviegoers free popcorn in two sizes that was either fresh or stale. What they found suggests we eat based not on taste but on size. In the two groups given fresh popcorn, those given the larger size ate nearly 50 percent more. What is more troubling is that among those given stale popcorn, the group who got the larger size ate nearly a third more! People eat more food when it is offered, even if it tastes bad (Wansink and Kim 2005).

In another study, the same team gave one group of participants a regular bowl of soup and the other group a trick bowl that self-refilled. The participants eating from the self-refilling bowl ate nearly 75 percent more soup but did not perceive themselves as eating more, nor did they report feeling more sated. Again, this research suggests that people feel full based not on the amount consumed but on the amount of food on the plate (or in the bowl). We are using our eyes, not our stomachs, to determine when we are full (Wansink and Kim 2005)!

It has been shown in several studies that eating while watching television leads both children and adults to eat more than if they were not watching television. It seems that people are not as attentive to how much they are eating when they are distracted by the TV. In a study in which the researchers varied the amount of TV time for a group of normal-weight 8- to 12-year-olds, they found that the kids who watched 50 percent more television than what they were normally accustomed to ate 250 more calories and exercised less than they ordinarily did (Epstein et al. 2002). TV may take time away from physical activity, and the content of TV often contains messages, subtle and overt (like advertisements), encouraging consumption.

ENERGY OUT

Just as some research has suggested that the differences in the prevalence of obesity across countries are due to diet, other research suggests that the higher prevalence of obesity in some countries is mostly due to lower physical activity levels. So is it energy out and not energy in?

The energy-out portion of the energy balance equation is comprised of three elements: the BMR, energy expended in physical activity, and the thermic effect of food. The BMR (or resting metabolic rate) comprises approximately 60 percent of daily energy expenditure. It is the energy expended while at rest to keep vital organs and systems operating. BMR is determined by the fat mass, fat-free mass, age, and sex of the individual. It decreases with age and loss of lean body (muscle) mass and is higher in men. The thermic effect of food changes with foods consumed. As the percentage of energy from carbohydrates (versus fat or protein) increases, energy expenditure increases, but the effect is very small and very hard to measure. The thermic effect of food is about 10 percent of daily energy expenditure. In sum, this means that between 60 and 80 percent of energy expenditure isn't something we can easily modify. The remaining portion of energy expenditure, about 400–800 calories per day, is intentional physical activity. Energy expenditure (EE) is a simple equation:

$$EE = BMR + \text{thermic effect of food} + \text{physical activity EE.}$$

Energy expenditure varies between individuals because of several factors. Individuals with a bigger body size have higher levels of energy expenditure because it takes more energy to move a larger body than a smaller body the same distance. Individuals who have lost weight often expend less energy as well. Different types of muscle fiber also burn calories differently, and training can alter the distribution of muscle fiber type. Gender also plays a role in energy expenditure.

Over the last century, Americans have seen a decline in manufacturing and agricultural jobs and a corresponding increase in professional and services jobs. This means fewer people are active at work. At the same time, more people are driving to work (instead of walking or walking to take public transportation), and with the expansion of the suburbs, the amount of time spent commuting has increased. Despite these changes, the amount of leisure time Americans have has actually increased, thanks to energy-saving devices. And while people perceive themselves as having little free time, the average American actually spends nearly four hours a day watching television! Part of the increase in leisure time comes from the decrease in time spent on domestic and household tasks, but the gains in free time have largely been allocated to more TV time. Interestingly, research shows that the body's metabolism is 15 percent lower watching television than lying in bed!

The landscape for energy expenditure in the United States has changed in other ways during the evolution of the obesity epidemic. In the late 1970s and early 1980s, cities and towns across the country began facing budget shortfalls. One of the first things to get cut as school budgets were slashed was funding for physical education (PE). To decrease costs, schools began exempting some students from PE. Other schools began cutting PE to allow more time for traditional classroom instruction in order to improve scores on the standardized tests that were increasingly administered in science and math. By the end of the 1980s, Illinois was the only state requiring daily PE. Many school districts justified the cuts by noting the rise in private sports clubs and teams for kids. Unfortunately, these were a luxury largely limited to middle- and upper-class children living in the suburbs. By privatizing fitness, urban and low-socioeconomic status children, those least likely to have access to safe places for recreation, were left most at risk of being sedentary.

At the same time, parents were being offered a rather convenient babysitter —cable television. With loads of options to keep children occupied, busy parents could get things done and know children were "safely" at home. Not surprisingly, the more TV kids report watching, the less active they are. This is a matter of both choice and options. Compounding the TV-exercise trade-off is the fact that children's television programming is filled with ads for snack foods largely void of nutritional value, leaving kids full of messages to eat more and to eat more of foods that are less healthy.

We talked about temporal changes in the calories we take in, and we can see there have also been changes in energy expenditure. Whether or not the amount of time spent in leisure-time physical activity has changed is the subject of some dispute. The government sponsors several studies that measure physical activity in the population, and while one suggests few changes have occurred over time, another suggests the amount of time spent exercising has declined.

GENETICS

There are rare instances of obesity being caused by a mutation in a single gene. These cases of obesity are early onset (where "early" means the first days or months of life) and are generally also accompanied by neuroendocrine abnormalities. The genetic mutations typically occur in genes associated with making or regulating the hormones leptin and melanocortin.

Studies of twins and people who have been adopted clearly show that obesity has a hereditary component. That is, twins who have grown up separately have been found to have similar weights and fat deposits as adults. And when adopted children grow up, they end up having the same pattern of obesity as their biological parents.

Common obesity (the kind we all think about when we hear the word) has a genetic component, but it is likely linked to mutations in more than one gene, and genes are only one part of the cause. Common obesity is also caused by nongenetic factors. The way that genes and lifestyle interact to cause obesity is like baking bread: the genetic mutations are the basic ingredients like the flour, eggs, milk, and butter, and the lifestyle factors are like the yeast that triggers the dough to rise. Genetic factors likely explain between 20 and 60 percent of obesity (though estimates range from 10 to 90 percent!), with other factors (age and lifestyle factors like diet, exercise, and the other factors discussed in Chapter 5) explaining the remaining portion. Loos and Bouchard (2003) have proposed a model that hypothesizes about the contributions of the environment and genes on obesity (see Figure 3.4).

For those with genetic obesity, the environment has little effect. Similarly, there are likely some individuals whose genetic profiles leave them largely "immune" from the effects of the environment. This is the person we all seem to know who can eat and eat and eat, never exercise, and never gain weight. For the rest of the population (the vast majority), the environment has an effect, but how large an effect is a function of genes.

The genetic mutations that have been identified as associated with obesity are also associated with an increase in hunger and lower levels of inhibition.

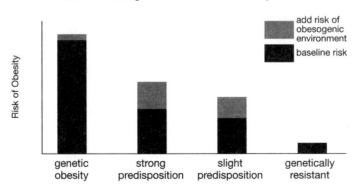

Figure 3.4. Effect of obesogenic environment on obesity risk [After Loos and Bouchard 2003/Jeff Dixon].

For example, an individual may have a genetic mutation in which the body sends no signal or only a weak signal to the brain to say the stomach is full or that there is enough fat stored in the body. As a result, the individual keeps eating because the brain is not receiving the signal to tell the person, "Enough!" Or the mutation may be in the brain, where a receptor is not functioning as it should. In this case, the body is sending a strong signal of "Enough!" but the particular receptors in the brain are malfunctioning and not receiving the signal to stop eating.

You may have heard people talk about a *thrifty gene hypothesis* for obesity. The hypothesis was put forward by James Neel in the 1960s and says that as man was evolving, selection was high for genes that promoted fat storage (storing energy as fat rather than as glycogen in the muscle). Such a metabolic profile would be advantageous in times of food scarcity as the individual could draw on his or her large fat stores and survive longer than individuals without such a genetic mutation. In an environment of abundance, like the one most Americans live in, such a genetic mutation would be detrimental, as those fat stores are not called upon and so continue to grow. The theory has great appeal, but the scientific evidence to support it isn't all that strong. While immigrant studies show the rapid rise in obesity when populations move into a calorie-dense environment (like the United States), data from genetic studies are lacking. Few candidate genes or gene-environment interactions to support the thrifty gene theory have been identified.

Many potential genetic determinants of obesity have been identified, including genes that control fat metabolism, but they have not been consistently linked to common obesity. Identifying genes that might cause obesity is challenging because it requires large samples of individuals, extensive testing, and the ability to collect data before and after obesity arises. It is clear that in order to fully understand obesity from a genetic perspective, researchers will have to explain more clearly how the environment interacts with genetic mutations.

DISPARITIES

What do these causes say about the disparities between groups in the prevalence of overweight and obesity that were mentioned in Chapter 2?

The reasons for the differences between groups are not entirely known. There are many factors that may contribute to ethnic disparities in overweight and obesity. And these factors may influence one another in complex ways. Research has suggested that neighborhood characteristics, socioeconomic factors (e.g., income, education), neighborhood safety, cost and accessibility of healthy foods, and lack of physical activity are some of the factors that may contribute to the differences in the prevalence of obesity between different ethnic groups. We'll talk in more detail about these in Chapter 5. Briefly, the occupants of low-income neighborhoods may consume foods from a convenience store if a grocery store or supermarket is not close by. These stores are more likely to sell junk foods high in fat and sugar. Thus, the people in that neighborhood may consume foods that are energy dense and nutrient poor because that is what is most readily available to them. There is also some indication that cultural differences are at work. For example, Hispanic mothers may encourage their children to eat more because they may think that children who are plump are healthier (Kimbro 2005). Researchers have done some interesting research to examine how the prevalence of obesity among immigrants changes over time. Individuals who move to the United States and Canada tend to become more overweight or obese the longer they live in their adopted countries.

WHAT DOES THIS MEAN FOR OBESE KIDS?

If the same factors can cause obesity in kids and adults, and obesity does have a genetic component, does that mean obese kids are destined to be obese adults? Not necessarily, but it does increase the odds. A conservative estimate is that childhood overweight predicts 40 to 60 percent of adult obesity (Freedman et al. 2005a). Weight patterns in childhood and adolescence tend to continue into adulthood. Obesity in childhood increases the risk of high blood pressure, respiratory problems (including asthma and sleep apnea), glucose intolerance, hyperinsulinemia, insulin resistance, and high cholesterol. And as we'll discuss later, obesity in adulthood increases the risk of many diseases, including cardiovascular disease, type 2 diabetes, and some cancers. In order to study this question, some researchers have examined BMI at certain ages throughout childhood and adolescence in order to predict the risk of becoming obese in adulthood.

A study that tracked 2,400 children for 17 years in rural Louisiana found that obese children (BMI $\geq$ 95th percentile) were more likely to be obese adults (BMI $\geq$ 30). There were racial differences in the proportion of obese children who remained obese in adulthood. When broken down by race, 65 percent of white girls and 84 percent of black girls remained obese in adulthood. The reason for these differences is not clear, but the authors of the study hypothesized that blacks may experience a larger BMI increase between childhood and adulthood. The results of this study did show that black girls and overweight black boys experienced higher annual increases in BMI in childhood and adolescence as compared to white girls and overweight white boys (Freedman 2005a).

Another study from the same group of children in Louisiana found that BMI-for-age in childhood and triceps skinfold thickness (SF) were associated with adult BMI and the mean of adult subscapular and triceps SF. This study is notable not only because it showed that childhood BMI and SF predicted adult BMI and SF but also because it demonstrated the future risk of obesity due to overweight even at a very young age. For example, two- to five-year-olds who were obese (BMI-for-age $\geq$ 95th percentile) were over four times as likely to become overfat adults (mean SF in the upper quartile) as compared to two- to five-year-olds with a BMI-for-age < 50th percentile (Freedman et al. 2005b).

The BMI values of children and adolescents at the 75th, 85th, and 95th percentiles according to the Centers for Disease Control and Prevention BMI-for-age growth charts are also related to overweight and obesity at age 35. One study found that overweight or obesity in childhood and adolescence increased the probability of becoming an overweight or obese adult. And age seems to make a difference. That is, older overweight or obese adolescents are even more likely to become obese adults. For example, for girls with a childhood or adolescent BMI at the 95th percentile from age 5 to 12 years, the probability of adult obesity was between 40 and 59.9 percent. The probability of adult obesity for a girl in the 95th percentile from age 12 to 20 years rose to $\geq$60 percent. For boys at the 95th percentile, the probability of adult obesity was between 20 and 39.9 percent from ages 4 to 12 years, 40 to 59.9 percent from ages 12 to 17 years, and $\geq$60 percent from ages 17 to 20 years (Guo et al. 2002).

Preventing childhood and adolescent obesity is urgently needed, and intervening earlier in life may prevent suffering in both childhood and adulthood. In order to combat pediatric obesity, researchers are recommending six levels that should be considered for further investigation and action: family, schools, health care, government, industry, and media (Pietrobelli et al. 2008). We'll talk more about the specifics of what is being done in Chapter 5.

Understanding the causes of obesity provides a foundation for understanding the detrimental consequences of the condition and what strategies might work for preventing and treating overweight and obesity.

4

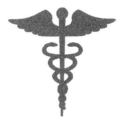

Complications of Obesity

"[Obesity researchers say that] when it comes to obesity, nothing is as straightforward as it may appear."

(Kolata 2002)

Every day there are headlines in the news about the health consequences of obesity. "Obesity and High Cholesterol in Children Are Seen as Warning of Heart Disease," heralded *The New York Times* on November 12, 2008. "Diabetes Strikes Younger and Younger," warned *USA Today* the very next day. "Chronic Adult Ailments Find New Victims in Obese Kids," lamented the *Chicago Tribune* in March 2008. In 2002, the U.S. surgeon general stated that obesity would overtake tobacco as the leading cause of preventable death in America. Obesity has been shown to increase the risk of developing type 2 diabetes, heart disease, some cancers, and liver and gallbladder disease. In addition, obese people suffer from higher rates of sleep apnea, mood disorders, and impaired quality of life. Obese children and adolescents are being diagnosed with chronic illnesses that were once seen only in adults! Illnesses such as type 2 diabetes, fatty liver, hypertension, high cholesterol, and sleep apnea are increasingly being diagnosed in children. This has resulted in increased hospital stays for this age group. Pediatricians and public health officials are scrambling to address the problem. While not everyone can agree on the best way to solve this problem, everyone agrees that this trend is extremely alarming.

An early death is not the rule for all obese people. The truth is that researchers don't yet have all the answers to the complications stemming from obesity. Some researchers question whether obesity is a disease or a symptom of disease. In short, we still have a long way to go in investigating the many effects obesity can have on humans. In this chapter we will discuss the most common potential health complications that stem from obesity.

MORTALITY

Being overweight or obese can lead to an early death. The estimated number of U.S. adults who die each year from obesity-related causes ranges from 112,000 to 325,000 (Allison et al. 1999; Flegal et al. 2005). The life expectancy of obese adults is lower than for nonobese adults. Researchers at the American Cancer Society undertook one of the largest studies on the topic of obesity and death from all causes. They studied over 1 million healthy, nonsmoking adults from 1982 to 1996. The results were clear: Regardless of age, the higher the body mass index (BMI), the greater the risk of death. Men who had a BMI between 23.5 and 24.9 kg/m^2 and women who had a BMI between 22.0 and 23.4 kg/m^2 had the lowest risk of death. People who had the highest BMIs had two times the risk of dying prematurely as compared to people who had the lowest BMIs (between 18.5 and 24.9). When the researchers looked at black men and women separately, they found that those who had the highest BMI did not have significantly increased risk of death (Calle et al. 1999). Some studies have also found that having a very low BMI increases the risk of death.

Due to better treatments of infectious disease, better sanitation, and better public health overall, the life span of people living in the United States has been steadily increasing over the last 200 years. At the turn of the 20th century, the average life span in the United States was 49.2 years. In 2005, the life expectancy at birth of someone living in the United States was 77.8 years (Kung et al. 2008). In fact, the U.S. Census Bureau projects that the average U.S. life expectancy will be 82.6 years in the year 2050. However, some researchers argue that we could begin to see a leveling off or even a decrease in the life span of Americans. One study conservatively estimated that obesity has the potential to shave two to five years off the average life span of children (Olshansky et al. 2005).

Most of the studies that have examined the relationship between obesity and premature death consisted of mostly or only white participants. It is clear that more work needs to be done to better understand the risk of premature death in other ethnicities. This is important because as was discussed in Chapter 2, the prevalence of obesity is higher in racial and ethnic minorities. Obesity is known to cause low levels of long-term inflammation of tissues throughout the body. This is known as systemic inflammation. Research has shown that elevated abdominal obesity is related to systemic inflammation. Adipose tissue (fat cells) produces proinflammatory molecules that travel throughout the body. In fact, adipose tissue is considered by the medical community to be an endocrine organ since it produces so many molecules and chemicals. The body's inflammatory response is also an immune response and is meant to protect us when we are injured or have an infection. For example, if you cut your finger, you can tell that the body's inflammatory response is working because you feel pain and heat and notice swelling and redness at the injury site. This is a sign that inflammatory molecules in the body are working to kill bacteria that may have gotten into the cut, cordon off the affected area so that bacteria cannot spread further into healthy tissue, and allow the healing process to begin by attacking any damaged tissue around the cut. However, sometimes the inflammatory response can work against the body. In the case of autoimmune diseases, such as lupus, the inflammatory response is exaggerated and healthy tissue is damaged. Obesity-related diseases such as heart disease, diabetes, and cancer are thought to be related to inflammatory chemicals in the body.

There is evidence that abdominal obesity contributes to the risk of death from all causes. Waist circumference is one way to measure abdominal obesity. A study of over 45,000 U.S. women found that those with the highest waist circumference ($\geq$35 inches) had significantly increased risk of death as compared to women with the lowest waist circumference (<28 inches) (Zhang et al. 2008).

So does losing weight mean obese people will live longer? Several researchers have studied this question by having people report their own weight loss. The results showed that obese people who lost weight actually had increased mortality rates! How could this be? The answer is not clear, but some scientists think that the way that some people are losing weight may not be safe. For example, people are drawn to fad diets, unregulated herbal supplements, or unhealthy behaviors to lose weight, such as bulimia. The best way to study the question regarding the effect of weight loss on mortality rates is to enroll people in a study where they utilize safe methods of weight loss and are monitored by research staff. Other researchers suggest that people may be losing weight, but they are not losing fat. A few studies that used calipers to measure skinfold thickness (fat composition) have shown that fat loss led to reductions in mortality, but weight loss was related to increased mortality. This is an area that needs more research to rule out the effects of weight loss that may be occurring due to an undiagnosed illness.

Examining the relationship between obesity and death from all causes does not tell the whole story about the effects of obesity on society. There are thousands of people who suffer the disabling consequences of obesity in the form of type 2 diabetes, cardiovascular disease (CVD), cancer, sleep disorders, and psychological distress. Not only do these complications affect the individuals experiencing them, but also they take a toll on their families. The expense of treating these complications also places a huge burden on the health care system and society at large.

RISK OF TYPE 2 DIABETES

As the number of people categorized as obese has risen in the United States, so too has the number of people with type 2 diabetes. According to national data, in 2007 about 23 million Americans had diabetes (7.8 percent of the population) and 1.6 million were newly diagnosed with the disease. Of the 23 million Americans with diabetes, 17.9 million were diagnosed cases and 5.7 million were undiagnosed. Between 1980 and 2006, the number of people in the United States diagnosed with diabetes tripled from 5.6 million to 16.7 million (Centers for Disease Control and Prevention [CDC] 2008a; see also Figure 4.1). National studies show that the number of people suffering from diabetes is increasing in both adults and children. Statistics also indicate that 57 million people in the United States age 20 or older suffer from a condition called prediabetes. In prediabetes people have elevated blood glucose levels, but the levels are not high enough to classify them as diabetic. However, prediabetics have a high likelihood of developing full-blown diabetes within 10 years.

Diabetes is a disorder of metabolism. Normally, when we digest food it is turned into glucose that then moves into the bloodstream to allow cells to function. The pancreas excretes the hormone insulin, which processes the glucose and allows it to be absorbed by cells in the body (muscle, liver, fat) and used as energy. People with diabetes have a problem processing the glucose in the blood. In type 1 diabetes, the pancreas does not produce enough insulin to allow the glucose to be absorbed by cells in the body. In type 2 diabetes, the cells in the body don't respond to the insulin. This is called *insulin resistance*. In either case, glucose is left in the blood and is not absorbed by the tissues in the body such as the liver, muscle, and fat tissue. Having excess glucose in the

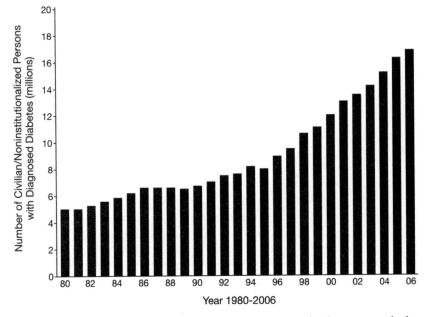

Figure 4.1. Number (in millions) of civilian/noninstitutionalized persons with diagnosed diabetes, United States, 1980–2006 [After CDC/Jeff Dixon].

blood is known as *hyperglycemia*. All the extra glucose in the bloodstream can lead to cardiovascular disease, kidney problems, blindness, nerve damage, and poor blood circulation, which can lead to amputations of toes and feet. The body senses that glucose is not being absorbed and tries to fix this by having the pancreas produce even more insulin, resulting in a condition known as *hyperinsulinemia*.

Treating diabetes involves monitoring blood glucose levels in order to address hyperglycemia. Some oral hypoglycemic medications can be used to increase insulin sensitivity and promote the response of beta cells in the pancreas to glucose. One of the downsides of using hypoglycemic drugs is that they promote weight gain. Depending on the severity of diabetes in an individual, injections of insulin are needed. Usually this happens when other measures to control the amount of glucose in the blood have failed. In diabetics, it is important to closely monitor blood sugar and administer the proper amount of insulin. For example, injecting too much insulin may lead to hypoglycemia.

Obesity is the main risk factor for type 2 diabetes. According to the CDC, 90–95 percent of people diagnosed with diabetes are diagnosed with type 2 diabetes. About 80 percent of people with type 2 diabetes are overweight. Studies have shown that as BMI increases so does the risk of type 2 diabetes. One study of men indicated that having a BMI ≥ 35 kg/m^2 conferred over 40 times the risk of developing diabetes as someone who was considered normal weight (BMI < 25) (Chan et al. 1994). Weight gain is also associated with the risk of developing type 2 diabetes. Sixty percent of newly diagnosed cases of diabetes can be directly attributed to weight gain (James et al. 2003). Female nurses who gained 7 to 10 kg (15.4 to 22 lb.) after the age of 18 had two times the risk of type 2 diabetes as compared to nurses whose weight remained stable (Colditz et al. 1995).

How Does Obesity Contribute to the Development of Type 2 Diabetes?

Science has demonstrated that the accumulation of body fat leads to higher levels of insulin in the bloodstream in both men and women because, in part, being obese causes the tissue in the body to be insulin resistant. Studies have shown that having fat around the waistline (central adiposity) leads to greater insulin resistance and therefore results in increased hyperinsulinemia. The mechanism through which obesity leads to insulin resistance is complex and not fully understood, but it is believed to relate to the way in which adipose tissue influences metabolism. Adipose tissue releases free fatty acids and bioactive proteins (adipokines), which may affect insulin action (Westphal 2008). Recent research also indicates that inflammation may play a role in the development of insulin resistance. White blood cells, called *macrophages*, are part of the immune response and are located in bone marrow. In the example of the cut finger we discussed earlier in this chapter, macrophages would attack any bacteria that entered the body through the cut. Sometimes macrophages enter adipose tissue or liver tissue and release chemical messenger molecules called *cytokines*. Cytokines have been found to cause tissue they come in contact with to become insulin resistant. Researchers from the University of California, San Diego, fed mice a high-fat diet, but in one group of mice they manipulated the cells in the bone marrow and disabled the process that leads to inflammation in macrophages. Normal mice would be expected to become obese, develop inflammation, become insulin resistant, and develop type 2 diabetes. However, no insulin resistance or type 2 diabetes developed in the mice for which the inflammation process was blocked (Solinas et al. 2007). The results of this study may be important for humans because if a drug could be developed to block the inflammatory process, then it is possible that type 2 diabetes could be prevented. However, extrapolation of findings from studies in mice to humans should be done with caution as many other differences between the species may result in failure to replicate the finding.

It worries doctors that the rates of obesity among children and adolescents have increased because it has been accompanied by an increase in the diagnosis of type 2 diabetes in this population. Studies have shown that children and adolescents who are overweight produce more insulin, and as mentioned above, eventually the cells in the body become less sensitive to the insulin. This eventually leads to type 2 diabetes. Because overweight and obesity are affecting more and more children and adolescents, there is more type 2 diabetes in this group. This form of diabetes was historically seen only in adults. Now, 45 percent of all diabetes cases currently diagnosed in children are type 2 diabetes!

Frequency of fast food consumption increased the risk of weight gain and the risk of developing insulin resistance in a study of young adults. Both white and black participants who ate two or more meals per week from fast food restaurants gained 4.5 kg (about 10 lb.) and had two times the rate of insulin resistance as compared to participants who ate fast food meals less than once a week (Pereira et al. 2005). This study showed that frequent fast food consumption may increase the risk of developing obesity and type 2 diabetes by influencing weight gain and insulin resistance. We'll talk more about fast food restaurants and obesity in Chapter 5.

Despite reports from hospitals that type 2 diabetes is increasingly being diagnosed among youths, there is little national data on the prevalence of type 2 diabetes in children and adolescents. The SEARCH for Diabetes in Youth study was started in 2000 by the National Institutes of Health (NIH) because they recognized that data on how many kids in the United States have diabetes and how this number may have changed over time do not exist. In order to understand the burden of diabetes among young people in this country, surveillance data are important. According to the SEARCH for Diabetes in Youth study, approximately 3,700 people under 20 years old were diagnosed with type 2 diabetes between 2002 and 2003 in the United States (Writing Group for the SEARCH for Diabetes in Youth Study 2007).

We know that some ethnic groups have a higher risk of developing diabetes. The Pima Indians of Arizona and other American Indian tribes have the highest number of new cases of diabetes each year, followed by Mexican Americans. African Americans, Asian Americans, and Pacific Islanders also suffer disproportionately from type 2 diabetes. Researchers have suggested some reasons why Mexican Americans experience higher rates of type 2 diabetes. Studies show that compared to nondiabetics, diabetic Mexican Americans have a higher weight at a younger age, gain weight more rapidly after age 18, and have more trunk fat relative to leg fat (Joos et al. 1984). This is important because longer duration of obesity and abdominal obesity are both related to increased risk of type 2 diabetes.

Leading a sedentary lifestyle is also a risk factor for developing diabetes. There is evidence that weight loss alone or combined with physical activity can decrease the risk for developing type 2 diabetes by decreasing glucose levels in the blood and improving the insulin sensitivity of body tissue.

Diabetes Prevention Program (DPP)

Does weight loss help to prevent type 2 diabetes? In 2002, researchers published the results of an intervention study that examined weight loss among over 3,200 overweight people who had prediabetes in 27 centers around the United States (Knowler et al. 2002). The researchers studied the participants for an average of three years. Forty-five percent of the participants in this study were minorities. People were randomly assigned to one of four groups. Group 1, called the "lifestyle intervention group," received individual counseling to eat a modified diet (low fat, fewer calories), do 150 minutes of exercise each week, and change their behavior. The people in the lifestyle intervention group were told to aim to lose 7 percent of their body weight and keep the weight off. Another group of participants took metformin, an oral diabetes drug. A third group was given a placebo, a pill containing no drugs. A fourth group started out taking a drug called troglitazone, but the researchers had to stop this study arm soon after the study started because it was found that the drug caused liver damage.

Regardless of gender or ethnicity, the lifestyle intervention group ended up decreasing their risk of developing diabetes by 58 percent as compared to the placebo group. In the lifestyle intervention group, those over the age of 60 decreased their risk by 71 percent as compared to the placebo group. The group who took metformin decreased their risk of developing diabetes by 31 percent. However, the drug was most effective among people between the ages of 25 and 44 who were a minimum of 60 pounds overweight (BMI $\geq$ 35). In the placebo group, 11 percent developed diabetes compared with 7.8 percent in the metformin group and 4.8 percent in the lifestyle intervention group. In summary, the DPP demonstrated that lifestyle changes such as weight loss and exercise can prevent or delay the onset of type 2 diabetes in overweight prediabetics. The drug metformin was also helpful in decreasing the risk of developing diabetes, but the results were not as dramatic as the effect that the lifestyle intervention had on risk. These results are great news for the 57 million Americans who have prediabetes because it shows that they can delay or prevent type 2 diabetes.

Look AHEAD: Action for Health in Diabetes

Recognizing that obesity and type 2 diabetes increase the risk for cardiovascular disease, mortality and suffering, researchers at the National Institute for Diabetes and Digestive and Kidney Diseases division of the NIH started a study in 2001 that will continue until 2012. They are examining the long-term effects of weight loss and exercise in overweight people with type 2 diabetes. The study is called Look AHEAD: Action for Health in Diabetes. The study is being conducted in 16 different areas of the United States and includes an ethnically diverse population of over 5,000 volunteers. For four years, half of the participants will have ongoing contact with study counselors, receive a program of increased physical activity, and eat a portion-controlled diet (reduced calorie, moderate fat). The other half of the participants will attend an educational program on diabetes and nutrition. All the participants will be followed until 2012, and the researchers will then examine the long-term health impact of the intensive weight-loss intervention on CVD in obese people with type 2 diabetes (Ryan et al. 2003). The results of this project will provide essential information to doctors and public health officials regarding strategies that may work to sustain long-term weight loss.

RISK OF CANCER

Researchers estimate that 14–20 percent of all cancer deaths in the United States can be blamed on being overweight or obese (Calle et al. 2003). This means that if all the adults in the United States could keep their BMI under 25 during their lives, 90,000 deaths per year from cancer might be prevented. In addition, higher body weight has been shown to be associated with higher death rates for particular types of cancer. Obesity also increases the risk of developing cancer. The World Cancer Research Fund and the American Institute for Cancer Research (WCRF and AICR) published a report in 2007 after reviewing all the scientific research on weight and cancer. The experts who wrote the report said that the scientific evidence is convincing that body fatness contributes to cancers of the esophagus, pancreas, colon and rectum, female breast (postmenopausal), endometrium, and kidney (renal cell) (WCRF/ AICR 2007). In fact, there is a dose-response relationship between BMI and risk of these cancers. That is, as BMI increases, so does the risk of each of these cancers. Although studies have examined the association of weight and risk of other cancers (e.g., liver and thyroid), the results are not consistent enough to draw firm conclusions. In other words, some studies may have shown a positive relationship between thyroid cancer and obesity, and other studies showed no relationship.

Normally, cells in the body grow and multiply in a controlled manner. Cancer develops when a mutation occurs and results in uncontrolled growth of the cells in the body. Cancer cells lack or have turned off the cell mechanisms that tell them to stop replicating. As a result, these cells accumulate and a tumor grows. Cancer cells also have the ability to spread from their point of origin to other parts of the body.

How Does BMI (Body Fatness) Cause Some Cancers?

Researchers have implicated excess body fat, which is measured by BMI in most studies, as a convincing cause of esophageal, pancreatic, colorectal, postmenopausal breast, endometrial, and kidney cancers (WCRF/AICR 2007). Body fat has a direct effect on the body, stimulating production of hormones and growth factors that in turn stimulate cell growth and discourage cell death. Fat also stimulates the inflammatory pathways, which can contribute to uncontrolled cell growth in cancer.

In the case of esophageal cancer, frequent gastroesophageal reflux, when the acid from the stomach goes into the esophagus, is a risk factor for the cancer. Gastroesophageal reflux often occurs in individuals who have a high BMI. The irritation and inflammation associated with the reflux has been shown to exacerbate the inflammatory process and contribute to the development of esophageal cancer (WCRF/AICR 2007).

Why Is Abdominal Adiposity Considered an Independent Risk Factor for Some Cancers?

Research has shown that abdominal adiposity is a convincing cause of colorectal cancer independent of BMI. It has been proposed that abdominal adiposity increases risk by increasing levels of circulating estrogens and reducing insulin sensitivity. The WCRF/AICR report points to abdominal obesity as a probable cause of pancreatic, postmenopausal breast, and endometrial cancers. A study of U.S. women showed that risk of death from any type of cancer increased with increasing abdominal obesity (Zhang et al. 2008).

Aside from body fatness, weight gain in adulthood is considered a probable cause of postmenopausal breast cancer. For every 11 pounds in weight gained in adulthood, the risk of developing postmenopausal breast cancer increases by 5 percent (WCRF/AICR 2007). As previously stated, increased weight is associated with higher levels of circulating hormones. Among postmenopausal women, increased hormones, particularly estrogen, circulating in the blood are problematic because estrogen has been shown to increase the risk of breast cancer. The main source of estrogen in premenopausal women is the ovaries. In postmenopausal women, the ovaries no longer produce estrogen, and estrogen is produced by the fat tissue. As a result, obese postmenopausal women are subjected to prolonged estrogen exposure, thereby increasing their risk of breast cancer. Weight loss in postmenopausal women has been shown to reduce the risk of breast cancer (Eliassen et al. 2006). It is thought that the reduction in risk seen with weight loss is due to decreases in the levels of circulating estrogen combined with the interplay of other hormones that may promote breast cancer.

The WCRF/AICR (2007) report stated that there is convincing evidence that body fatness and abdominal fatness are related to increased risk of colorectal cancer. As discussed in the section on diabetes in this chapter, the accumulation of body fat leads to higher levels of insulin and glucose in the bloodstream. The excess body fat that results from obesity also leads to higher levels of leptin and growth factors circulating in the bloodstream. Insulin, growth factors, and leptin can all promote the growth of cancer cells in the wall of the colon (WCRF/AICR 2007). Researchers have linked higher levels of plasma glucose and higher levels of insulin and leptin in the blood to an increased risk of colorectal cancer (Giovannucci et al. 1995; Stattin et al. 2004). Most studies investigating the relationship between obesity and colorectal cancer have found that association is stronger in men than women. This may be because men typically gain weight around their abdomen and women gain weight in their hips and thighs. Central adiposity leads to increased hyperinsulinemia. The resulting excess insulin in the blood may stimulate cancer cells in the colon to grow. Weight gain is related to risk of colon cancer in men. A study of over 46,000 men found that weight gain since age 21 and weight gain in the past 10 years was related to an increased risk of colon cancer (Thygesen et al. 2008).

Body fatness has been shown to decrease the survival of women with breast cancer and increase the risk of recurrence. One study found that the rate of mortality from breast cancer in very obese women (BMI $\geq$ 40 kg/m^2) was over three times higher than the rate in very lean women (BMI < 20.5 kg/m^2) (Petrelli et al. 2002). It has been shown that severely obese women are about half as likely to be screened for breast cancer as normal weight women. The reasons for this are not clear, but it has been suggested that obese women may find getting a mammogram particularly uncomfortable. Alternatively, it may be that it is harder to detect breast cancer in obese women due to excess breast tissue, which may make it harder to find a lump.

CARDIOVASCULAR DISEASE

CVD is the number one cause of death in the United States. It kills more people than the number who die from cancer, chronic lower respiratory diseases, accidents, and diabetes combined (Thom et al. 2006). In 2003, over 910,000 people in the United States died from CVD, according to the

American Heart Association. That statistic amounts to one death every 35 seconds. The risk of CVD increases with age. Men experience higher death rates from CVD than women. Unfortunately, the risk of developing heart disease may, in part, be inherited from our parents. While some of the risk of CVD is in our genes, there are several lifestyle factors that contribute substantially to risk, including high blood pressure (hypertension), high cholesterol, high BMI, physical inactivity, diabetes, and smoking.

There are clear racial and ethnic disparities in CVD health. For example, African American and Mexican American women experience more of the risk factors for CVD than whites. The rate of hypertension in African Americans is the highest in the world! As a result, African Americans have one and a half times the rate of heart disease death of whites.

CVD includes coronary heart disease (CHD), stroke, congestive heart failure, and sudden cardiac death. Obesity increases the risk of all the illnesses that fall under the umbrella of CVD by increasing risk of hypertension, high blood lipids (i.e., cholesterol), and insulin resistance. Dyslipidemia is a disorder of lipoprotein metabolism. It is characterized by high levels of total cholesterol, elevated LDL (bad) cholesterol, low HDL (good) cholesterol, elevated triglyceride concentrations, or a combination of abnormal levels of any of these three lipoproteins. This imbalance can lead to atherosclerosis, which is often described as "hardening of the arteries" and is a major risk factor for CVD. Dyslipidemia is an independent risk factor for CVD. Obesity increases the risk of developing CVD, and one of the ways it impacts CVD is via its detrimental effect on blood lipid levels. Recent evidence has shown that obesity may act to cause CVD through the formation of blood clots and inflammation. It is estimated that more than 45 percent of the 9.3 million cases of CVD can be attributed to obesity (Wang and Dietz 2002).

In addition, researchers now believe that obesity has a direct, independent effect on the development of CHD, although the mechanism is not clear. The Framingham Heart Study followed 5,209 people living in Framingham, Massachusetts, for 26 years and found that obesity is an independent risk factor for CHD (Hubert et al. 1983).

Being overweight or obese also increases the risk of death from CVD. A study of over 1 million people in the United States found a significant increase in the risk of death from CVD in men whose BMI exceeded 25 kg/m^2 and in women whose BMI exceeded 26.5 kg/m^2 (Calle et al. 1999).

There is a strong relationship between obesity and high blood pressure, a strong risk factor for CHD. Results from the landmark Framingham Heart Study showed that the blood pressure in obese participants was twice the blood pressure of normal-weight participants (Hubert et al. 1983). In addition, hypertension is seen more often in people who have had a longer duration of obesity.

Obesity actually causes structural changes in the heart. Obese people have an increased total blood volume because they have more tissue (fat, muscle, and skin) that needs to be nourished by the blood supply. As a result, the heart has to work harder to pump blood to all this tissue. Scientific studies have shown that due to the increased blood volume in the obese, there is increased filling of the left ventricle of the heart and increased cardiac output. The increased filling puts stress on the walls of the left ventricle, and the heart compensates by stimulating growth of the heart wall. The growth of the heart wall causes it to thicken, and this hampers the ability of the ventricle to contract, so less blood is pumped out. How much the wall of the left ventricle thickens and grows depends on the degree of obesity and the length of time a person has been obese.

New research has suggested that obesity causes the body to be in a state of chronic low-level inflammation. Markers of inflammation in the blood have been identified as predictive of CHD.

Abdominal Fat

In 1947, Professor Jean Vague from the University of Marseille in France published a scientific article in which he observed that patients with hypertension, diabetes, or CVD typically had more body fat around the abdomen (android obesity). He also noted that patients who had more of a female distribution of body fat (gynoid obesity) did not have these health problems. Thus, he suggested that the location of body fat was more important than total body fat in the development of health problems. It took over 30 years for the scientific community to follow up and confirm on his observations with rigorous scientific studies (Fairburn and Brownell 2005).

Having body fat that is concentrated around the abdomen is now a known risk factor for CVD. People who have a high concentration of fat around their abdomen have been shown to have dyslipidemia, insulin resistance, and hypertension as well as systemic inflammation. These are all independent risk factors for the development of CVD. Abdominal fat has been shown to be a risk factor for heart attack and stroke in men. Increasing waist circumference is also related to increased risk of death from CVD among women. Even normal-weight women (BMI 18.5 to 25.0 kg/m^2) with abdominal obesity are at increased risk of dying from CVD (Zhang et al. 2008). In both women and men, higher waist-to-hip ratio or waist circumference is related to increased risk of CVD. Central adiposity has been shown to contribute to the promotion of CHD. As a result of the evidence linking waist circumference to CHD, some researchers have proposed that it should be considered a "vital sign" that should be measured at doctors' appointments just like blood pressure and body temperature.

Weight Gain

Moderate weight gain in adulthood has also been associated with increased risk of hypertension, stroke, and CHD. A study of female nurses between the ages of 30 and 55 years found that the more weight a woman gained in adulthood, the higher her risk of CHD. In fact, a weight gain of 11 to 19 kg (24 to 42 lb.) after age 18 conferred two times the risk of CHD as compared to women who maintained a stable weight (Willett et al. 1995). What is striking about this study is that the women were all considered "normal" weight, with a BMI in adulthood between 20 and 24.

More and more research is indicating that CVD has the potential to become a pediatric illness (Belluck *The New York Times* Nov. 12, 2008). For example, research suggests that being overweight as an adolescent increases the risk of developing CVD. Studies have also shown that being moderately overweight as a teenager can lead to an increased risk of death from CVD before age 66, no matter what the person weighed as an adult (Must et al. 1992).

A study of overweight children between 5 and 10 years old in Louisiana found that 61 percent had at least one risk factor, such as high blood pressure, high cholesterol, and elevated insulin levels, for CVD. This is not a normal age to start seeing these risk factors emerge. In the past, these risk factors did not manifest until adulthood.

One recent study found that the arteries of children between the ages of 6 and 19 who were obese or had high blood pressure were as thick as the arteries of a typical 45-year-old (Belluck *The New York Times* Nov. 12, 2008)! In light of the growing body of research on CVD in children, pediatricians are especially worried that the health of American youths has been compromised by obesity.

CARDIA

The Coronary Artery Risk Development in Young Adults (CARDIA) study tracked risk factors for CVD in over 5,000 African American and white young adults (ages 18 to 30) from Birmingham, Alabama; Chicago, Illinois; Minneapolis, Minnesota; and Oakland, California. The study started in 1985 and is ongoing. Participants periodically answer questions about their diet; take a treadmill test to determine their fitness; have their blood drawn to measure cholesterol and glucose; and have their weight, height, and blood pressure measured.

Researchers from the CARDIA study have published several notable scientific articles that significantly increased scientific knowledge about CHD outcomes. One analysis used coronary artery calcification as a proxy for atherosclerosis. This analysis demonstrated that participants who had the highest central adiposity in young adulthood had double the odds of developing atherosclerosis at an early age (ages 33 to 45) as compared to participants who had the lowest level of central adiposity (Lee et al. 2007). The study also demonstrated that greater waist circumference or waist-to-hip ratio in 1985–1986 was associated with greater odds of coronary artery calcification in 2000–2001. Lifestyle choices at one time in life can affect outcomes much later, highlighting the importance of establishing healthy choices early in life.

When an obese person with high blood pressure presents at a doctor's office, the doctor will typically recommend weight loss and exercise. Surprisingly, few studies have examined the effect of weight loss on CVD. This may be due to the fact that obesity has only recently been recognized as an independent risk factor for CVD. However, there have been many studies of the effect of weight loss on risk factors for CVD. Weight loss in overweight and obese people has been shown to reduce blood pressure, blood glucose, insulin, blood lipids, and markers of inflammation. However, even if a patient manages to lose weight, studies have shown that it is very difficult to keep the weight off, and most people gain the weight back.

Studies of weight loss in overweight or obese people with high blood pressure have shown that losing about 5 percent of total weight can decrease blood pressure. However, even if this new weight is maintained, over time the reduction seen in blood pressure starts to get smaller. That is, the blood pressure levels start to rise again. Thus, the implication of weight loss on CVD risk requires more research.

ASTHMA

Both asthma and obesity have increased simultaneously in adults and children for several decades. However, researchers are unsure as to whether asthma is part of the cause of obesity or vice versa. It could be that having asthma causes people to exercise less, and as a result, they become obese. Alternatively, obesity may contribute to or exacerbate asthma. The scientific evidence relating obesity to asthma is inconsistent. Several studies have suggested that being obese could be a risk factor for developing asthma. However, some studies have not found obesity to be a risk factor for asthma. What is clear is that we need more research in order to better understand the relationship between obesity and asthma. Let's take a closer look at what we do know.

Asthma is a long-term inflammation of the lungs that causes the airways (breathing tubes) to be swollen and very sensitive. Because the airways are inflamed, the tubes leading into the lungs are narrower. People who suffer from asthma often have episodes of wheezing (a whistling sound when they breathe), feel their chest tightening, and have difficulty catching their breath. A lot of substances in the air, such as pollution and pollen, can irritate the lungs of a person with asthma. If the lungs are irritated, the body responds by tightening up the muscles around the airway, swelling in the airway may become worse, and cells in the airway may create mucus. All of these responses make it more difficult for a person to take air into his or her lungs.

The causes of asthma aren't well known. Several hypotheses exist for how obesity may increase the risk of asthma. Asthma may be more of a problem in obese people because of mechanical issues. In obese people there is more weight on the chest, more fat surrounding the chest wall, and more blood flowing around the lungs to nourish the extra tissue. In other words, the extra weight pressing on the lungs makes it harder to breath, and less air reaches deep into the lungs.

As mentioned above, inflammation of airways is the very definition of asthma. Some researchers have suggested that the chronic, low-level systemic inflammation throughout the body that accompanies obesity could explain why asthma is more of a problem for obese people. It could make conditions favorable for asthma to develop in the first place, or the extra inflammatory molecules circulating in the blood of an obese person may worsen existing asthma. Gastroesophageal reflux is also related to the risk of asthma. And as mentioned previously, gastroesophageal reflux often occurs in individuals with a high BMI and has been shown to exacerbate the inflammation.

In a study in which people breathed into a machine that measured the level of inflammatory agents in their lungs, the researchers found that levels of nitric oxide (a proxy for airway inflammation) did not increase with increasing BMI. The authors suggested that this may mean that the mechanical explanation for the increase in asthma among the obese is more likely than the systemic inflammation hypothesis.

The California Healthy Kids Survey of over 470,000 5th-, 7th-, 9th-, and 11th-grade students conducted between 2003 and 2005 found that the rate of doctor-diagnosed asthma increased with increasing BMI regardless of ethnicity or gender. The risk of having asthma increased even in kids who were in the 45th to 55th percentile of BMI, not just overweight and obese kids (Davis

2007). Some studies have indicated that after puberty, the relationship between asthma and obesity is stronger in girls than boys.

Some studies show that weight gain increases the risk of asthma, and others have shown no increased risk. Few studies have been conducted to examine the effect of weight loss on asthma, and they included only whites. Overweight or obese adults with asthma who lost weight either through diet modification, behavioral changes, and/or bariatric surgery had fewer asthma symptoms, used less asthma medication, utilized fewer health care services, or demonstrated better lung function (Ford 2005). Unfortunately, no studies have adequately examined weight loss and asthma in children.

SLEEP DIFFICULTIES

Obesity is thought to cause sleep difficulties because of the problems that excess weight poses to the lungs. Excess weight makes it difficult for the lungs to expand and contract. Increased fat around the abdomen also makes it hard for the lungs to expand and take in a full breath. Increased fat around the neck increases pressure on airways, especially when lying down.

Sleep apnea is a common complication of obesity. In Greek, apnea means "without breath" (http://www.sleepapnea.org). People with sleep apnea typically snore loudly and stop breathing for at least 10 seconds at a time between 5 and 30 times each hour. The process of the airflow stopping and starting so often results in shallow breathing that prevents the person from experiencing deep sleep. When someone stops breathing, the brain sends signals to arouse the person to start breathing again. As a result, people who suffer from sleep apnea are extremely tired during the day because they have had frequent interruptions of their sleep. The sleep that they do get is not restful because it keeps getting interrupted. If you have ever seen someone with sleep apnea stop breathing and then struggle to start breathing again with a loud snore, it is quite unnerving. Of course, most people don't know they have this problem because they are asleep!

A BMI > 30 is common among people with sleep apnea. Researchers estimate that 40–90 percent of obese subjects are affected by obstructive sleep apnea (OSA) (Arias et al. 2005). OSA occurs when the airway is blocked. Lack of muscle tone in the upper airway means that there is soft, floppy tissue that collapses in the back of the throat. When a person tries to take a breath when he or she is lying down, this floppy tissue actually blocks the airflow.

Sleep apnea affects children and adolescents too. Researchers examined U.S. hospital records between 1979 and 1999 in order to measure the level of obesity-related diseases that doctors were diagnosing in kids between the ages of 6 and 17 years. The diagnosis of sleep apnea increased dramatically in that time period. In fact, over that time, the total number of diagnoses of sleep apnea increased 175 percent (Wang and Dietz 2002)!

Recent research has shown that not having enough sleep may actually be a risk factor for obesity, especially among children (Patel 2008). How does a lack of sleep lead to weight gain and obesity? Some researchers have proposed that a lack of sleep leads to increased hunger by impacting the hormones that regulate hunger. In addition, if you aren't sleeping, you have more time to eat, so this leads to increased food intake. Lack of sleep obviously causes fatigue, which makes a person less likely to do physical activity. There is also some suggestion that lack of sleep has an effect on the ability of the body to keep a steady temperature (thermoregulation), and although the mechanisms are not fully understood, researchers have suggested that this may lead to reduced energy expenditure.

If sleep apnea goes on for months and years, it has been shown to lead to hypertension, heart failure, and psychological consequences. Obese people have a higher risk of developing sleep apnea, and sleep apnea leads to sleep deprivation, which has been shown to be a risk factor for obesity. The obesity-sleep/sleep-obesity relationship is a self-perpetuating cycle. Sleep deprivation has been shown to lead to auto accidents, less productivity in adults at work, and problems for children in school. There is some evidence that weight loss can alleviate sleep apnea.

QUALITY OF LIFE

The study of obesity and quality of life has expanded significantly in the last 10 years. Research suggests that obesity has a detrimental effect on quality of life. Quality of life in overweight and obese subjects is typically measured by querying self-reported physical function, psychological function, and social function. People who are obese report a lower quality of life. The excess weight an obese individual carries may reduce his or her ability to function physically due to pain or difficulty moving. For example, the extra weight that the joints of an obese or overweight person bear may lead to pain and osteoarthritis. The intolerance, prejudicial treatment, and general stigma associated with being obese may impact emotional health and create more difficulty in social situations. Extremely obese study subjects have reported suffering from severe psychological stress.

Quality of life among obese people is lower for women than men, decreases with increasing BMI, and is worse among those who are suffering from another illness at the same time. We do know that some obese people experience tremendous personal suffering due to the stigma and discrimination they face. In addition, obese people may experience feelings of guilt. Thus, people who repeatedly attempt and fail at dieting in order to lose weight have a lower quality of life.

Obese people may rate their quality of life as low because they are suffering from other obesity-related chronic diseases, such as diabetes. However, research suggests that obesity is related to quality of life independently of other illnesses. One survey found that the percentage of people reporting excellent health decreased with increasing BMI in whites, blacks, and Hispanics who were not suffering from any other chronic condition (Okosun et al. 2001).

A study of over 40,000 female nurses followed for four years found that increasing BMI and gaining more than 20 lb. during the study period, regardless of their starting weight (BMI), predicted decreased daily physical functioning, decreased vitality, increased bodily pain, and decreased feelings of well-being (except among women age 65+) (Fine 1999). In general, weight loss of 20 lb. or more among overweight and obese women in this study was related to an increase in physical functioning, increased vitality, and decreased bodily pain. In this study the feelings of well-being in women over the age of 65 years were not impacted by weight gain. It has been suggested that the stigma against obese people may be directed less at the elderly (Rand and Wright 2000).

Unfortunately, obese people face discrimination, or "fat bias." It has been found that obese people are discriminated against when they apply for jobs, and they may earn less money. In addition, people report having a negative attitude toward obese people.

Children who are overweight have been found to have low self-esteem and are not happy about their ability to perform physical tasks. Overweight kids are bullied and teased about their physical appearance. Of course, the negative attitudes toward kids who are overweight make them feel badly about themselves. In a study that set out to understand children's attitudes about obesity, the researchers showed the children silhouette images of people. The children used words like "ugly," "dirty," "lazy," and "dumb" to describe the silhouettes of obese people (Wardle et al. 1995). Indeed, Tiffany King, the girl we met in Chapter 3, wrote about the unwanted attention her physical appearance attracts in her application essay to the weight loss camp: "Sometimes, if I'm walking down the street, I can hear people talking about me and staring at me" (Saul 2008).

A lot of the research on weight and quality of life has been undertaken among obese people who seek treatment for obesity. In general, people who are seeking treatment for obesity have lower quality of life and higher rates of anxiety and depression as compared to those who have not sought out treatment. Young adults and adolescents seeking treatment for obesity often have problems with anxiety and eating disorders. In the Swedish Obese Subjects (SOS) study, a study of over 1,700 patients surgically treated for weight loss, obese participants rated their quality of life as low as or lower than people suffering from advanced cancer or severe chronic pain. The level of pain those seeking treatment for obesity report is similar to the level of pain that patients with migraine headaches report. And their psychological well-being is worse than patient groups who have suffered paralysis less than two years after a spinal cord injury, have rheumatoid arthritis, or have been diagnosed with cancer within the last two to three years (Sullivan et al. 1993).

Patients from the SOS who sought treatment for obesity report that taking part in social activities in public places is very troubling to them. Both men and women rated trying on or buying clothing as the most troubling, followed by swimming in public, visiting a restaurant, and traveling on vacation, compared to nonobese people from the general population (Östman et al. 2004). In addition to the aforementioned psychosocial problems, obese patients seeking treatment had more symptoms of anxiety and depression than nonobese subjects from the general population (Karlsson et al. 2003). Just the idea of being perceived as overweight was shown in one study to influence general health, vitality, and physical function more than actual BMI (Burns et al. 2001).

Some research has shown that losing weight improves the quality of life of obese people. For example, more weight loss resulted in greater improvements in quality of life among obese subjects in the SOS study who were surgically treated for obesity. Six months postsurgery, those who lost 22.05 lb. to more than 66.14 lb. had dramatic improvements in quality of life. Four years postsurgery, researchers concluded that in order to maintain the improvement in quality of life, the subjects had to maintain their 20–25 percent weight loss from surgery (Östman et al. 2004). Ten years postsurgery, researchers found that those who maintained weight loss reported better health-related quality of life. Unfortunately, the positive effects of weight loss on health-related quality of life population-wide are reduced because so many surgically treated patients regain weight (Karlsson et al. 2007).

Body image is how a person perceives or judges the appearance of his or her body in terms of its size and shape. It is a multidimensional issue because society, cultural attitudes, and personality are just some of the components that factor into the image a person has of his or her body. Obese people frequently report dissatisfaction with their body size. Studies of body dissatisfaction in obese subjects have shown that dissatisfaction increases with increased

BMI. However, the obesity-body dissatisfaction relationship varies depending on a person's perception of his or her own weight. That is, people who perceive that they are more overweight than they actually are will have lower satisfaction with their bodies. These studies have also shown that the degree of dissatisfaction is generally greater for whites as compared to African Americans. Why does this difference exist? There is speculation that cultural differences may account for the racial and ethnic differences in body satisfaction, especially among African American women. That is, higher body weights may be viewed more positively in the African American culture. In addition, some research has suggested that to some, beauty is not so one-dimensional as to be defined by body size and weight alone. Personal style and presentation along with body size and weight are factored in when black female adolescents consider their overall appearance (Parker et al. 1995). In a study of body size estimation, white overweight or obese participants had higher body dissatisfaction because they had an exaggerated view of their body size and underestimated what an "ideal" body size would look like, as compared to African American participants (Williamson et al. 2000). Other studies have shown that regardless of ethnicity or gender, the higher a person's BMI, the more he or she overestimates his or her actual body size.

Results from the CARDIA study of black and white young adults demonstrated that regardless of BMI, age, or education, blacks were more invested in appearance (e.g., attach more importance to appearance and grooming) and more satisfied with their appearance as compared to whites. Women, regardless of race or ethnicity, attached more importance to physical appearance than men. Both black and white women had more dissatisfaction with their body weight or shape than men. Overweight black women were more satisfied with their appearance than white women. However, obese black and white women had similar body size dissatisfaction. And black men reported the highest satisfaction with their physical appearance, while white women reported the lowest satisfaction (Smith et al. 1999).

Weight loss would seem to be the answer for people who have a poor body image. And studies have shown that weight loss does improve body image. However, researchers have found that the relationship between weight-loss and body image is complicated by factors such as individual weight-loss goals, personality, and how highly an individual regards physical appearance.

Although a lot of knowledge has been gained from the study of obesity in relation to quality of life in the past 10 years, this field of research is still fairly new, and future studies may help to clarify the mechanisms by which obesity impacts quality of life, especially among children and teens. For example, we need to learn more about how ethnicity, gender, education, and economic status play into the relationship between weight and quality of life. In addition, more work needs to be done to understand the effect of weight loss, weight gain, and abdominal adiposity on quality of life.

FIT VERSUS FAT

So being overweight is bad for your health, right? Surprisingly, despite all the data we've presented, not all research says so. Let's take a look at two debates currently ongoing in the research community.

In 1999, a group of researchers combined data from five big studies in the United States and estimated the number of deaths attributable to obesity (Allison et al. 1999). More than 80 percent of the deaths were in obese individuals (BMI $\geq$ 30 kg/m^2). The study authors estimated that between 280,000 and 325,000 deaths could be attributed to obesity. However, other researchers felt that the methods used to analyze the data in that study may not have been correct, and the errors would have overestimated the number of deaths due to obesity (Flegal et al. 2004). One of their concerns was that the individuals excluded from analysis in the previous study might be those at highest risk of death and most likely to die from causes unrelated to obesity. Thus, excluding these individuals would overestimate the percentage of deaths attributable to obesity. Other researchers defended these exclusions as necessary because individuals with lower BMIs are sometimes suffering from undiagnosed illnesses that lead to weight loss (like some cancers), and including them falsely overestimates the death rate in the nonobese population (Willett et al. 2005). Similarly, smokers tend to weigh less, so the lean group in any population is a mix of smokers, those with diseases, and healthy individuals. The critics of the 1999 study did their own analysis in a different data set. They found that obesity was associated with excess deaths, though many fewer than the first analysis had suggested (just under 112,000), and that overweight was not associated with death at all (Flegal et al. 2005). Later, looking at specific causes of death, they found that being overweight was associated with a *decreased* risk of death from causes other than cancer and CVD and was not associated with risk of death from cancer or CVD (Flegal et al. 2007). Obesity did increase risk of cancer death for cancers thought to be associated with obesity. The concern with this analysis is that it didn't disentangle the different sets of individuals comprising the lean population, making it possible that disease, which may ultimately cause death, also caused the weight loss (something researchers call *reverse causation*). This debate continues to go on as researchers debate the most appropriate way to analyze the data.

In an equally heated debate that continues to go on, some researchers have questioned whether it is really obesity that is the most important risk factor for excess mortality, arguing that fitness is more important. These researchers studied a population of men, measured their BMI and their cardiovascular fitness, and followed them for eight years. Men who were overweight and unfit had the highest mortality rates. But men who were overweight and fit were less likely to die than men who were normal weight and unfit (Lee et al. 1999). They subsequently found similar results in women. But a different group of researchers found something different in an analysis of another data set (Hu et al. 2004). Looking at self-reported physical activity, BMI, and death over a 20-year follow-up period, these researchers found that physical activity reduced the risk of death, regardless of BMI. Women who were overweight and active did have a lower risk of death than those who were sedentary. But being physically active did not erase the increased risk of mortality that came with being overweight or obese. At every physical activity level, heavier women were more likely to die than leaner women. Subsequent studies have examined the joint effects of exercise and obesity on other health outcomes, including CVD and diabetes (Lee et al. 2009; Weinstein et al. 2008). These studies indicate that both are important risk factors. Fitness can attenuate, but not eliminate, the risk that being overweight poses for diabetes, and those who are overweight and inactive remain at highest risk. Similar findings have been found for CHD.

SUMMARY

Scientific research has shown that the storage of excess fat leads to disease and ultimately death. It is clear that BMI, abdominal fat, and weight gain are culprits in the risk of developing diabetes, CVD, and cancer. There is evidence that physical activity and weight loss can decrease the risk of having a heart attack, improve blood lipid levels, and decrease blood pressure. Obesity also has negative side effects on psychological health. With a long list of harm done by obesity, the need for effective prevention and treatment programs is apparent.

5

Prevention and Treatment of Obesity

As noted in Chapter 1, there is a long history of strategies to treat obesity as well as an extensive literature on how to prevent it. In this chapter, we focus on a few of the most popular areas in the prevention and treatment of obesity, both in the lay and scientific press. We'll review lifestyle interventions focusing on diet and physical activity. We'll also visit new research indicating that the physical and social environment can affect body weight. Finally, we'll examine medication and surgery options for obesity treatment.

LIFESTYLE

Changing our diet or physical activity level is what most of us are thinking of when we talk about losing weight or trying not to gain weight. Many approaches to both have been tried independently and together. We'll detail some of the more common approaches to weight loss and obesity prevention in adults and children. Why do we focus on changes in what we eat and what we do? Research has shown that people who gain weight do smaller amounts of vigorous physical activity (or none at all), watch more television, and snack more.

Dietary approaches to weight loss are extensive and the subject of much debate. Unfortunately for advocates of the most popular modern approaches, the best research we have to date suggests that each diet works about the same in helping individuals achieve long-term (at least one year) weight loss. Some diets work better for short-term weight loss, but everyone eventually achieves about the same amount of weight loss regardless of approach. Until the 1990s, much of the focus in the weight-loss literature and media was on low-fat diets. Weight Watchers, the DASH diet, and the diets advocated by the American Heart Association and American Cancer Society are all low-fat diets. They suggest adherents get no more than 20–30 percent of their calories from fat. These diets are also typically high (55–60 percent of calories) in carbohydrates. Several randomized trials of the low-fat diet have been conducted. In a randomized trial, participants enroll and are then assigned at random to the diet of interest, in this case a low-fat diet, or a control arm. Typically, the control arm receives usual medical care or a less-intensive intervention. An example would be the intervention arm receiving individual counseling on following a low-fat diet and the control arm receiving some general pamphlets on weight loss or eating healthy. Very low-fat diets ask adherents to consume no more than 10 percent of calories from fat. The Ornish and Pritikin diets are examples. These diets also discourage eating high amounts of refined carbohydrates. A 2003 study found that low-fat diets were no better than any other diet for long-term weight loss (Astrup et al. 2004; Klein 2004). The "Mediterranean" diet is a moderate-fat diet with about 25–40 percent of calories from fat. This approach focuses on the types of fat consumed, promoting monounsaturated fats, like those in olive oil, over saturated fat, like that in butter. It also promotes consuming high amounts of omega-3 fatty acids, a fat found in high quantities in fish but in low quantities in red meat.

An alternative approach is to focus on protein and carbohydrate consumption instead of fat. High-protein diets advocate consuming 25 percent of calories from protein. The Zone diet is an example of this approach. The theory behind high-protein diets is that protein has a higher satiating effect; thus, a high-protein diet is better than a high-carbohydrate diet because individuals will feel more full and eat less overall. Low-carbohydrate diets, like the South Beach and Atkins diets, advocate consuming little to no carbohydrates. These diets also promote the satiating quality of protein. They theorize that when the body doesn't take in glucose (found in high amounts in many high-carbohydrate foods), blood glucose levels drop and the body metabolizes fat for the glucose. The body uses glucose as the primary fuel for its cells. Thus, the hypothesis is that these diets lead to greater fat loss. Research has suggested that individuals on low-carbohydrate diets may lose more weight in the short term (six months later) than those on low-fat diets, but in the long term (one year later), there is no difference (Ebbeling et al. 2007). Low-carbohydrate diets have raised several safety concerns. When the body doesn't take in carbohydrates, it doesn't get the glycogen it uses for fuel, and the only source of glycogen left is protein. Some of that comes from dietary protein, but some comes from the body tissue. This can lead to dramatic weight loss in the first few days of a low-carbohydrate diet from the loss of glycogen, protein, and water. Low-carbohydrate diets also put adherents at risk of ketosis, a high amount of ketones in the urine, resulting from a decrease in blood pH. This comes from the increase in ketone bodies that accompanies the fat breakdown and can be toxic. Individuals with a high fat and high protein intake, as those following the Atkins plan often are, are also at increased risk of gout. Gout is a buildup of uric acid in the joints resulting in inflammation. As was discussed in Chapter 4, many believe inflammation is a major contributor to several chronic diseases.

Dietary approaches to weight loss and weight gain prevention have focused not just on what foods we eat but also on how we eat. In the 1980s, nutritional research suggested that people who consumed the same number of total calories in more meals per day (six instead of three) would feel less hungry and perhaps, over time, eat less (Critser 2003, 39). The theory was that glucose and insulin levels would remain more stable this way. Unfortunately, the message was misunderstood or poorly executed, and many individuals ended up consuming three meals of the same size plus two or three additional snacks or meals, thus increasing their calorie consumption! As we'll see later, people are poor judges of how much they consume. There is also limited evidence that stable glucose levels lead to weight loss.

Interventions have also sought to provide tools to help individuals eat less, regardless of what they eat. Early efforts promoted calorie counting, but many individuals found this to be quite difficult, especially as the number of meals consumed outside the home increased. Approaches that have shown promise are those that focus on monitoring behavior. Individuals who write down what they eat and what activities they do tend to eat less and do more because the process of journaling makes them more aware of their consumption and energy expenditure. To that end, pedometers have shown promise as a physical activity–promoting tool by allowing users to see exactly how many steps they take each day. Other tools help users identify the portion sizes included in nutrition guidelines. A serving of meat is only the size of a deck of cards, but many chicken breasts and steaks sold in grocery stores and restaurants are nearly double that size. Pictures and plastic models of serving sizes may also help individuals control their total caloric intake. Aside from focusing on specific eating behaviors or exercise, research has shown that individuals who are most aware of their weight change because of regular self-weighing have success at weight loss, avoid weight gain, and maintain weight loss. Typically, this means weighing daily or weekly. However, studies that have attempted to intervene and increase self-weighing have had only modest success at helping participants achieve weight loss.

In the early 1990s, much of the focus in the weight loss and weight gain prevention community was on diet. Perhaps because these studies had only modest success, by the late 1990s, the focus had shifted to increasing physical activity. By the turn of the century, most experts agreed the greatest successes came from approaches that include both. More recent interventions seem to be focused on harnessing technology to address diet and physical activity. The interventions delivered by health researchers in the 1990s resulted in modest weight loss over the typical intervention period (four to six months), and a majority of these individuals maintained the weight loss one year later. The challenge is that these interventions were often quite costly and relied on highly trained research staff at universities and hospitals. Ultimately, the success of these programs may not be in long-term weight loss but in the prevention of typical adult weight gain.

In addition to delivering interventions to the general population, some research has focused on reaching adults in specific settings that might facilitate weight loss or weight gain prevention, like work sites, community health centers, and grocery stores. Others have focused on specific at-risk groups, like pregnant women, diabetics, menopausal women, or those at increased risk of heart disease. Often weight-loss programs succeed in changing behavior (diet or physical activity), but their success at changing BMI is less clear. In general, lifestyle interventions aimed at changing diet and exercise patterns have shown moderate success in the treatment of obesity, leading to changes in weight, body fat distribution, and risk factors for comorbidities including blood glucose and lipid levels. While these studies do achieve significant weight loss in the treatment as compared to the control group, the magnitude of the weight loss is often modest. In a study that pooled the results of several high-quality studies, the mean weight loss was only 7.9 lb. (Franz et al. 2007). Another found the mean weight loss was less—just 4.9 lb. (Galani and Schneider 2007).

The content of lifestyle interventions can vary widely, but they generally are comprised of programs that provide information on healthy eating and physical activity. This information can be delivered in printed materials or in group classes. Some programs offer individual counseling with a nutritionist or exercise specialist. Studies that focused on exercise could offer home-based or supervised exercise sessions. While supervised sessions (i.e., at a gym) may lead to greater initial weight loss, home-based programs appear more effective for long-term weight loss because they establish a sustainable pattern. Many individuals in gym-based interventions stop attending the gym when the study ends. Diet programs may prescribe a specific calorie or fat intake or may provide more general recommendations to "reduce fat," "reduce red meat intake," or "increase fruit and vegetable" consumption. Recommendations to include specific quantities might suggest that participants consume a specific number of servings of fruits and vegetables each day or allow the participant to determine the extent of change. Because of the great variability in the content of the programs, it is difficult to synthesize across studies and conclude what the single best approach or message is. More recent studies have moved away from counting calories or fat grams and focused on broader lifestyle changes, like cutting sugar-sweetened beverages or junk food. This is because research has shown that people who eat more fast food aren't physically active, watch more TV, drink more sugar-sweetened beverages, eat lots of sweets, eat away from home frequently, and eat lots of high-fat foods also weigh more.

Let's take a look at a typical behavioral intervention: Researchers enroll 20–40 individuals in a study and randomly assign half to the control group. The control group receives usual care (which may mean no contact), a delayed intervention (they get the same intervention as the other group, but when the study is over), or a less-intense intervention (mailed brochures instead of a tailored program). The intervention is delivered in a group setting and involves a series of lessons. In the past, there was often little evaluation of whether the lessons related the areas of a particular problem to the study participant or whether the individuals had mastered the skill before moving on to the next topic. Later interventions attempted to tailor messages to the individual more or use problem-solving skills in the group setting to provide individualization. The group typically meets weekly for 16–24 weeks and then has less contact. Intervention messages focus on self-monitoring behaviors, goal setting, nutrition education, physical activity education, changing the cues that trigger one to eat, and problem solving.

Many of the approaches to obesity prevention in children have focused on schools. A school-based intervention is the kid equivalent of a work-site obesity intervention. These studies often aim to change multiple behaviors at a single time. For example, in Planet Health, middle school students received lessons on diet and reducing TV time and counseling in gym class about increasing physical activity with the goal of decreasing the amount of time they were sedentary, increasing their physical activity, decreasing their fat intake, and increasing their intake of fruits and vegetables (Gortmaker et al.

1999). The intervention was tested for two years in 10 schools in the Boston area. Five schools received the curriculum (intervention), and 5 schools were monitored and did not receive the intervention (control). The prevalence of obesity in girls in the intervention schools decreased from 23.6 percent to 20.4 percent while the prevalence of obesity among girls in the control schools actually increased slightly. There was no change seen in the prevalence of obesity in boys in the schools. The intervention also succeeded in decreasing the hours of TV the participants viewed and increasing fruit and vegetable intake. The study provides an example of what often happens in obesity prevention or weight-loss programs. The participants successfully meet some of the study aims but rarely meet all of them. Interventions are rarely equally successful for everyone in the study. In this case, the prevalence of obesity in boys was unchanged. This reminds us that the same approach won't work for everyone but that successful approaches do exist. Studies may succeed in changing diet and physical activity, but that doesn't always translate into a change in body mass.

Weight-loss programs are delivered to kids as young as preschool students and on up to high school and college students. Some programs combine environmental and individual approaches, as was done in a study that provided both nutrition education and an overhaul of the school cafeteria options (Foster et al. 2008). Students and families received information about eating healthy, increasing physical activity, and decreasing TV time. The school also changed the cafeteria options to be in line with the messages given to families. The intervention reduced the number of students who became overweight and the total number of overweight students.

The factors that lead to weight loss are not always the same as those that are effective at preventing weight gain. Why is a focus on obesity prevention (preventing weight gain) important? Weight loss, as we've seen above, is HARD! In kids, the patterns developed in childhood are even harder to break as adults, so preventing habits that promote obesity in children has particular importance. The best approaches to obesity prevention in kids are similar to those outlined above, many of which were interventions for obesity prevention and treatment. The most successful studies are multifaceted—targeting school lunch, classroom lessons, vending machine options, and recreation time including both physical education (PE) and play. However, even this may not be enough, and larger population-level approaches, like policy changes to control marketing to kids and food labeling, will be necessary. Family-focused interventions are also of interest given the rise of obesity in both kids and adults (parents). These interventions are most likely to succeed when they are focused on obesity prevention specifically (versus changing diet and physical activity). Unfortunately, the best interventions are often resource heavy and intensive, requiring lots of time and money, which diminishes both their sustainability and dissemination potential.

The sharpest increase in the prevalence of obesity occurs in early adulthood. Unfortunately, adult weight gain is almost always fat, and that makes it even more dangerous for health. Efforts to prevent adult weight gain have shown mixed success. Many efforts in this arena have focused on high-risk groups—the weight that women gain during and after pregnancy and don't lose, menopausal weight gain, smoking cessation–related weight gain, and the typical weight gain that occurs after marriage. Lifestyle interventions have had modest success in the prevention of obesity among overweight individuals. Those that aim to prevent weight gain in general show less success. The most successful interventions are those that directly contact individuals and provide counseling on diet or physical activity. Studies in which participants are mailed informational materials or those that provide phone-based counseling have had little effect on weight gain prevention.

Research has consistently shown that physical activity can prevent weight gain and can prevent regain of weight following weight loss. The data are less clear that physical activity alone can lead to weight loss. Emerging high-quality data suggest that an hour of moderate-intensity activity a day is likely necessary to prevent weight gain in the long term. At a minimum, researchers agree that 30 minutes of daily physical activity are necessary for health promotion (Physical Activity Guidelines Advisory Committee 2008). Consensus is that 60–90 minutes are likely necessary to prevent regain (Institute of Medicine of the National Academies of Science 2002; Physical Activity Guidelines Advisory Committee 2008). Individuals who focus on all domains of physical activity appear to be most successful. This means increasing not just leisure-time physical activity but also physical activity at work, at home, and while commuting. This might be done by taking the stairs instead of the elevator, parking at the far end of the lot instead of closest to the door, and making work breaks a time to move around a bit.

PHYSICAL AND SOCIAL ENVIRONMENT

Environments that are thought to promote or produce obesity are called *obesogenic*. Instead of thinking about individual causes of obesity, we're talking about population-level causes. Swinburn and colleagues (1999, 180) describe it as "the sum of influences that the surroundings, opportunities or conditions of life have on promoting obesity in individuals or populations." An example would be our increasing dependence on cars, which has coincided with a shift to mall shopping, suburban living, and eating on the go. Intervening at the environmental or population level also requires a different set of approaches and tools.

Several features of the physical environment are thought to have an effect on obesity, including food availability, transportation availability, design, zoning, and architecture. For example, low-income neighborhoods have more fast food outlets and small bodega-style quick marts and fewer large grocery stores with fresh produce. As Americans increasingly live in the suburbs, we have less access to public transportation and are more likely to live in neighborhoods full of cul-de-sacs that don't promote walking to a destination. Most buildings are designed with elevators located front and center and stairwells relegated to the far corners, where they are often locked, poorly lit, and hard to find. Thus, even if individuals living and working in these environments wanted to adopt obesity-preventing diet and physical activity behaviors, the physical environment they live and work in works against them.

Why is living in a neighborhood full of fast food restaurants problematic? We know that individuals who eat at fast food restaurants frequently weigh more. We also know that individuals with diets high in fat and sugar (as most fast food is) weigh more. Fast food restaurants serve large portions of inexpensive food. Research consistently shows that the more people are served, the more they eat. Finally, we know that food availability is associated with food consumption: When more food is available, people eat more.

On the plus side, it is possible to intervene on a population level and have effects on obesity without individuals having to make any changes in their habits. For example, if potato chip manufacturers reduced the fat content in their regular chips from 35 percent to 31 percent, the population's dietary fat intake from potato chips would decrease by 10 percent (Swinburn and Egger 2008, 182). This seems a lot more feasible than a huge countrywide intervention aimed at reducing consumption of potato chips by 10 percent! Unfortunately, population-wide interventions often require the support of institutions and individuals who may not have the prevention or treatment of obesity as a primary goal. They also often involve payoffs that are many years away. Population approaches that aren't primarily focused on obesity can often have effects (positive or negative) on obesity. For example, as gas prices soar above $4 per gallon and concerns about global warming and climate change have become a key political and personal focus, more individuals may choose to take public transportation or personal transportation (walk, bicycle). Thus, physical activity can increase (an obesity prevention and treatment intervention) as a byproduct of concerns about the environment and economics.

To address neighborhood features that are obesogenic, there are a number of options that communities can embrace. Zoning laws have recently favored single-use districts (residential versus commercial versus industrial). Returning communities to areas of mixed use (picture the kind of communities in movies like *Pleasantville* and *The Truman Show*) promotes walking. These communities have shops just a few blocks from residential areas, so individuals living in them are more likely to walk than drive to shop and run errands. Existing communities of this kind tend to be urban and are often in low-income areas. However, the urban revitalization movement occurring in many cities may bring more people and diverse businesses to neighborhoods. Zoning laws can also be used to help prevent fast food chains from opening in an area or to encourage grocery stores to open in an area. Organizations like the Food Trust in Philadelphia work to bring grocery stores to lower-income neighborhoods. Communities can also change traffic laws to calm traffic and make roads safer for bicyclers and pedestrians. The advantage these approaches offer is that they affect both children and adults. The presence of parks and outdoor recreation areas is also associated with higher physical activity levels. Some communities are responding by converting abandoned train tracks into trails that community members can use for walking and bicycling.

Which communities are most likely to be obesogenic? Unfortunately, low-income and minority communities—those whose residents are at the greatest risk of overweight or obesity—are most likely to have features that are obesity promoting. These neighborhoods have fewer supermarkets, fewer places to be physically active, more fast food restaurants, higher crime rates (which people frequently report as a barrier to being physically active), and higher amounts of advertising for foods of limited nutritional value.

Workplaces can also endeavor to make environments more weight friendly. Companies are increasingly realizing this is in their interest as nonobese employees have higher productivity and cost the company less in missed days of work and health insurance premiums. Workplaces can be designed with easily located, open, and friendly stairwells. Employers are also subsidizing active commuting (bicycling, walking) and public transportation commuting. Worksite cafeterias are offering healthier choices. Some workplaces have also begun promoting active break times and active meetings.

Some companies have hired outside consultants to institute weight-loss programs for obese employees (*Newsweek* 2008 http://www.newsweek.com/id/143790 Author is Jerry Adler). The employees may receive a monetary reward for losing a certain percentage of body weight. Some obesity researchers argue that it is unfair and discriminatory and that obese individuals are an "easy

---

Lincoln Industries

Many companies are instituting wellness programs for their employees at work. CNN recently profiled a steel plant, Lincoln Industries, in Lincoln, Nebraska, that offers stretching before shifts, subsidized gym memberships, smoking-cessation classes, and classes on health and nutrition. The company views its wellness program as an investment with terrific returns. For example, they spend $400,000 a year on the program but save $2 million per year in health insurance costs due to the fitness of their employees. In the 16 years that the program has been in place, the president of the company has noted that workers are more productive, have higher morale, and submit fewer worker's compensation claims for injuries sustained on the job. The company does not punish employees who do not wish to take part in the wellness activities. Lincoln Industries rewards participating workers with a company-paid vacation to Colorado to hike a 14,000-foot mountain. In order to qualify for the reward, the workers must meet certain fitness goals and be nonsmokers. This year, 103 out of the 565 workers at the plant qualified for the reward.

---

target." They point out that what a person weighs is only one aspect of a healthy lifestyle. Why not reward employees for other healthy behaviors such as wearing a seat belt, reducing stress, or getting enough sleep? As obesity rates are expected to remain high, society will increasingly have more of these questions to grapple with.

Obesity is clearly a problem in developed countries such as the United States. Internationally, obesity rates have also been rising, and what is most worrying about this is that developing nations are beginning to face a double burden. That is, developing nations struggling to contain infectious diseases, such as AIDS and tuberculosis, and simultaneously having to manage the diseases that are complications of obesity will cause a crisis in the already fragile public health care systems of these developing countries.

Policy changes may also help change individual choices and social norms about obesity risk behaviors. New York City has been a trendsetter in this venue, pushing laws that ban trans fats and that require providing nutritional information in restaurants (Lueck and Severson 2006). Trans fats are found chiefly in partially hydrogenated oils and have been found to exert more negative health effects on blood lipids than other kinds of fats. In 2007, restaurants in New York were no longer allowed to sell foods with more than 0.5 g of trans fat per serving. In 2008, that was expanded to include baked goods and products with deep-fried batter. California followed suit in 2008 (Steinhauer 2008). Also in 2008, New York required restaurants with more than 15 locations to provide nutritional information for the food on their menus (Rivera 2007). The law affects only about 10 percent of New York restaurants. The idea behind the law is that if consumers know how many calories and fat are in items, they will choose a healthier item. Unfortunately, these initiatives are still new, so the long-term effects of them on obesity are unknown. Despite that, interest in them is spreading, and New York state is considering expanding the New York City initiative to the rest of the state (Hakim and Confessore 2009).

One of the most popular places for interventions on an obesogenic environment has been in schools. How can schools be obesogenic? In the 1980s and 1990s, schools were strapped for cash, and many began contracting with outside vendors to provide lunch to students (Critser 2003, 43). Unlike food prepared in the cafeteria, some of these vendors provided food in hallways or courtyards that fell outside the jurisdiction of the federal school lunch nutrition guidelines. Research showed that foods offered at these lunch cart venues had nearly double the portion size and calorie content of similar options served in the cafeteria (Critser 2003, 46). The beverage and snack industries also came into schools at this time and offered financial incentives to cash-strapped schools for exclusively stocking their product. Perhaps it is not surprising, then, that sweetened beverage consumption in children increased by 135 percent between 1977 and 2001 (Nielsen and Popkin 2004). In the last few years, parents, educators, and advocates have worked to change the food options offered in schools. Much of the focus has been on vending machines, where schools have limited the contents or availability of vending options. In 2004, 39 percent of schools had a policy to restrict the presence of foods (like vending and soda machines) that compete with healthy cafeteria options. However, nearly 90 percent of schools still offer competing foods. Of those, over 95 percent offer sugar-sweetened beverages, but only 45 percent offer fruits and vegetables (Centers for Disease Control 2005; Greves and Rivara 2006).

Schools and parent groups have also worked with communities to offer safe routes to school so that children can walk or bike to schools. As gasoline prices continue to rise, schools are increasingly supporting this option as they decrease the money they spend on transportation. Unfortunately, budget crunches also mean many schools are eliminating PE classes or curtailing the number of days per week that kids attend. Elementary school students attend PE class an average of 2.5 hours per week (Kramer and Daniels 2008). PE is important because research shows that students who attend PE more than two days a week in fifth grade were approximately 40 percent less likely to be overweight or obese as students attending less frequently (Veuglers and Fitzgerald 2005). Those students who do attend PE classes often don't get much activity as class time is devoted to instruction instead. Further limiting opportunities for active time in children and adolescents, many schools in times of shrinking budgets have cut funding for after-school programs, which often provide opportunities for kids to be active.

Another place to look for examples of what it takes to lose weight successfully is the National Weight Control Registry (NWCR). The NWCR began in 1994 when researchers from Brown University and the University of Colorado recruited men and women through magazine and newspaper articles. To be eligible to enroll, participants must have lost at least 30 lb. (13.6 kg), have maintained that loss for at least one year, and be at least 18 years old. Since the study started, new participants have been continuously recruited. The researchers are interested in the characteristics of successful long-term weight loss and weight maintenance. The registry is currently tracking over 5,000 individuals who have lost weight and maintained that weight loss. When they first enter the study, registry members complete questionnaires about their weight history and the behaviors and strategies that they used to lose weight and keep the weight off. Then registry members fill out yearly questionnaires that ask about changes in their weight and weight-related behavior. The ways registry members lost weight varied. About 45 percent reported losing weight on their own, and about 55 percent reported getting help through a commercial weight-loss program such as Jennie Craig, a doctor, or a nutritionist. What the registry members do have in common are their behaviors and strategies to keep the weight off. Registry members who were successful at long-term weight loss and maintenance have had an average weight loss of 73 lb. (33 kg) and have maintained the minimum weight loss of 30 lb. (13.6 kg) for an average of 5.7 years. How did they do it? Those who were successful ate a low-calorie, low-fat diet; frequently self-monitored their food intake (e.g., limited quantity, avoided fried food); weighed themselves frequently; and did high levels of physical activity (e.g., one hour of moderate-intensity walking per day). Successful weight-loss maintainers also report eating breakfast every day and maintaining a consistent eating pattern (eating regular meals on weekdays, weekends, and holidays), watching 10 hours or less of television per week, and eating limited fast food. Data from the NWCR indicate that maintaining weight loss may get easier over time. If the registry members maintained their weight loss for two to five years, the chance of long-term success increased greatly (Wing and Hill 2001; Wing and Phelan 2005).

Participants in the NWCR must exert significant effort and be ever vigilant in order to be successful at long-term weight loss. It is their consistent and persistent use of a combination of behaviors and actions over the course of many years that has led to their successful long-term weight maintenance.

The researchers who work with the NWCR acknowledge that the study results may not be generalizable to all overweight U.S. adults because the registry participants are about 77 percent female and 95 percent white. However, the NWCR is important because it has identified strategies for successful weight-loss maintenance that may be helpful to other populations.

MEDICATION AND SURGERY

While lifestyle modification alone, including diet, exercise, and behavioral therapy, is the preferred and primary treatment method for obesity, in cases where this fails, medication and surgery are often used as secondary treatments. Patients and their physicians must make a careful assessment of the risks and benefits of these treatment options, including that weight-loss failure is still possible. The success of surgical and drug interventions is dependent on the continuation of diet and exercise routines that target a healthy lifestyle. These interventions are currently recommended and in use for obese adults, while considerable debate remains about safe and effective use in the adolescent population.

Drug Treatment

Adults with BMIs greater than 30 kg/m^2 who have attempted weight loss through physical and dietary interventions but have not seen positive results qualify for treatment with antiobesity medication. If a comorbid condition, such as hypertension or diabetes, is present, then the qualifying BMI value reduces to 27 kg/m^2 and above (Bray 2002). Currently, two FDA-approved drugs, sibutramine and orlistat, are available for long-term treatment of adult obesity. A number of other drugs that have shown potential as effective weight-loss agents are under FDA review for safety and efficacy. Typically, diet pills and supplements that are available over the counter and directly marketed to consumers have questionable effectiveness and the potential for significant negative effects.

Antiobesity medications influence weight loss by reducing the patient's overall caloric intake. Medications ideally affect weight loss and weight maintenance in order to prevent regain. Medication is considered effective if the patient loses more than four pounds in the first month and achieves 5 percent weight loss at six months. If a patient experiences discomfort or harmful side effects or if comorbid conditions do not improve, drug use should be discontinued. Medications can produce varying side effects (Bray 2002).

Sibutramine (Meridia)

Sibutramine, also known as Meridia, effects weight loss by causing earlier satiety. Satiety refers to a feeling of fullness after eating, so sibutramine allows users to feel full after eating less food than they would normally (American Association for the Advancement of Science 2006). Sibutramine induces satiety by preventing the reuptake of monoamines, including norepinephrine, dopamine, and serotonin (Aronne 2002). Monoamines are a type of neurotransmitter in the central nervous system that chemically signals the body to modify a particular activity, in this case food intake. Since sibutramine prevents the monoamine uptake, it is more readily available to signal the neuron that causes satiety. Thus, less neurotransmitter release is required to reach satiety than under normal circumstances, and further food intake is prevented.

Sibutramine has been shown to be effective for weight loss and maintenance in placebo-controlled trials (Aronne 2002). It does, however, result in side effects, including nausea, dizziness, insomnia, dry mouth, and, most notably, increased systolic and diastolic blood pressure and pulse rate. This precludes any patients who already suffer from hypertension from taking the medication.

Orlistat (Xenical and Alli)

Orlistat is the generic name for the prescribed medication Xenical, which effects weight loss by decreasing the body's absorption of fat. Orlistat reduces fat absorption by inhibiting pancreatic lipase, an enzyme that normally permits the breakdown of fat for storage. As a result of decreased fat breakdown, fat can be excreted from the body with feces rather than absorbed, causing soft, oily stool during the initial months of use. Additional side effects are reportedly mild and gastrointestinal (GI) in nature and include incontinence, flatus, and abdominal cramps (Aronne 2002). Orlistat interferes with the absorption of the fat-soluble vitamins A, D, and E. As a result, individuals taking orlistat should also take vitamin supplements. To minimize side effects and increase the effectiveness, patients should consume a diet in which less than 30 percent of their daily caloric intake is from fat (Bray 2002). In addition to weight loss, orlistat can also cause a decrease in cholesterol levels and improve glycemic control in diabetic patients (Aronne 2002).

To determine if orlistat could be safely used over the counter, a recent study of consumer behavior was conducted (Schwartz et al. 2008). The study included participants from 18 pharmacies who were permitted to purchase a maximum of three packages of orlistat along with a reference manual and a personalized online weight loss plan focusing on diet and exercise. The small user population consisted primarily of female, Caucasian, 30–59-year-old individuals, the majority of whom said that they were mildly to severely overweight yet considered their baseline health to be good or better. Results were provided for the 237 (out of the original 703 consumers screened) who purchased and used the drug and partook in follow-up phone interviews at specified dates postenrollment. Positive results were seen in a number of categories, from routine diet and exercise practices to significant weight loss and customer satisfaction. In February 2007, the FDA approved orlistat in 60-mg doses as the first over-the-counter weight-loss medication for persons 18 years or older. Currently, the 60-mg pill is being sold as part of a new weight-loss package labeled "alli." The alli plan includes the 60-mg orlistat capsules, a variety of reference manuals, and online access to "myalliplan," a weight-loss plan adapted specifically for each registered alli user.

Clinical Trials

Clinical trials of long-term drug treatments for obesity reveal comparable weight-loss success with the two FDA-approved drugs, sibutramine and orlistat, as well as a third major player, rimonabant. Although rimonabant is approved worldwide, the FDA has not approved rimonabant for use as an antiobesity treatment. A meta-analysis combining the results of 30 different antiobesity drug trials (16 orlistat, 10 sibutramine, 4 rimonabant) found the drugs resulted in less than 5 kg of net weight loss (5-kg difference between the intervention group receiving the drug and the control group receiving a placebo) (Rucker et al. 2007). All studies included in the meta-analysis were double-blind, placebo-controlled trials, which means that neither the subjects nor researchers knew who was getting the actual medication and who was receiving the placebo, a control pill with no pharmacological effect. Twenty-seven of the 30 trials used were weight-loss trials with dietary interventions in addition to the drug administration, and all trials used the clinically common doses of each respective drug: 120 mg orlistat three times daily, 15 mg sibutramine once daily, and 20 mg rimonabant once daily. The majority of subjects were middle-aged, Caucasian women, with an average weight of 200 lb. The studies had high attrition rates, which means that a significant number of subjects left the study at some point, and were funded largely by the pharmaceutical manufacturer, which may mean the studies were more likely to find a positive result. Individuals taking the drugs reported adverse effects including GI distress with orlistat, increased blood pressure and pulse rate with sibutramine, and increased risk for psychiatric disorders with rimonabant. The studies found several positive results, including decreases in BMI, waist circumference, and triglyceride levels for all three drugs and decreases in blood pressure and improvement in diabetes comorbidity for orlistat and rimonabant.

Fen-Phen

The use of fen-phen for the treatment of obesity exemplifies the uncertainty in cardiovascular outcomes when using weight-loss medications. Fen-phen is the combination of two anorectics, fenfluramine and phentermine. Anorectics are drugs that suppress appetite and therefore reduce food intake in overweight individuals. Phentermine, fenfluramine, and dexfenfluramine were each approved by the FDA in 1959, 1973, and 1996 for separate use for the short-term treatment of obesity. Problems arose in the mid-1990s when the off-label use of phentermine in combination with either fenfluramine or dex-fenfluramine became increasingly common. *Off-label use* means that patients taking the medication and/or physicians prescribing the medication were not following FDA guidelines. The use of the fen-phen combo was not approved by the FDA but rather inspired by a 1992 published study suggesting that the combined use led to considerable weight loss over an extended period of time (Colman 2005). Long-term use of these anorectics in addition to dual usage had not been approved by the FDA, yet a trend of increasing use of the drugs in these ways occurred in the 1990s.

The transition to long-term use of anorectics in the mid-1990s led to sustained treatment with antiobesity medications (Stafford and Radley 2003). Dexfenfluramine was the only one that had received FDA approval for long-term treatment of patients with BMI > 30 kg/m^2 (or 27 kg/m^2 if a comorbidity was present), but the approval was for it alone, not in combination with phentermine. Still, clinicians noted a substantial increase in the use of fen-phen and dexfen-phen from 1995 to 1997 until reports of adverse effects were made public. After the Mayo Clinic reported valvular heart disease in 24 female fen-phen users on July 8, 1997, the FDA issued a public health advisory asking that health care professionals report any similar findings to the organization and received additional reports of heart valve disease for patients taking fen-fluramine or dexfenfluramine alone or in combination. No reports of valvular heart disease were received for patients taking phentermine alone. Valvular heart disease was indicated by leaky valves precluding normal heart function. It is common for affected individuals to be asymptomatic, or have no physical signs of their disease. The FDA requested that fenfluramine and dexfenflur-amine manufacturers voluntarily withdraw their respective drugs from the market and fen-phen consumers discontinue their use. The drug companies complied on September 15, 1997 (U.S. FDA 1997).

Market withdrawal of these two popular drug treatments led to a sharp decline in their use in the late 1990s. Consumers had generally ignored earlier warnings of adverse effects (Stafford and Radley 2003). In a population-based study of adults in six states who took prescription weight-loss pills between 1996 and 1998, researchers found that only one-third of fen-phen users had stopped taking the drugs after the FDA public health advisory, and a second third discontinued use after the market withdrawal (Blanck et al. 2004). This still means that one-third of users continued to use these drugs after withdrawal, indicating that patients were willing to take significant risks in order to take advantage of the potential weight-loss effects of the drugs. Although fen and dexfen are no longer available (as of 2004), phentermine remains available. Presently, most pharmacotherapy involves long-term use of sibutramine or orlistat, whose adverse effects, particularly cardiovascular, are still under study.

Other Drugs

Obesity treatment drugs can generally be classified according to their mechanism of action: to reduce food intake, alter metabolism, or increase energy expenditure. While orlistat is a preabsorptive drug that prevents fat from breaking down before it can be absorbed, metformin is a postabsorptive drug. It is effectively used to treat diabetes mellitus and has led to significant weight loss in double-blind placebo trials.

Drugs that increase energy expenditure include thyroid hormones, ephedrine, and caffeine. The use of thyroid hormones aims to increase metabolism in obese patients who are commonly thought to have a "low metabolic rate." In a six-month trial comparing ephedrine, caffeine, and a placebo, the three groups had similar weight loss, but a fourth group taking both caffeine and ephedrine had significantly more weight loss (Bray 2002). It is important to remember that none of these treatments, except sibutramine and orlistat, have received FDA approval for weight loss.

Adolescent Medication Use

Pharmacotherapy is not conventionally considered for the treatment of pediatric and adolescent overweight. Although sibutramine and orlistat are both in use among the adult population, only orlistat is FDA approved for overweight adolescents, 12 to 16 years of age, with BMIs in the 95th percentile for their age and gender. Orlistat can be made available to adolescents only through prescription; the over-the-counter forms available are approved only for adult use (Dunican et al. 2007). Recent studies indicate that sibutramine also has weight-loss potential in adolescents, but concern surrounding adverse cardiovascular effects has generally precluded FDA approval.

Studies of adolescent usage of orlistat have shown significant weight loss in some cases but in others have shown no difference between the drug and a placebo pill. Physicians have concerns about prescribing orlistat to adolescents as it can interfere with vitamin and mineral absorption, which could have significant effects on growth and maturation. Some studies have found no significant effects on calcium, phosphorous, magnesium, zinc, and iron balance, while others revealed vitamin deficiencies. As a result, the FDA recommends packaging a multivitamin with orlistat for patients 12 to 16 years of age (Dunican et al. 2007).

Clinical trials of adolescent usage of sibutramine showed significantly lower BMI, weight, and waist circumference. Some studies have found no difference in heart rate and blood pressure between those on sibutramine and those on a placebo while other studies have found that increases in diastolic blood pressure and pulse rate were noted for sibutramine patients. These trials generally involve a behavior change intervention in addition to the administration of medication (Doggrell 2006; Dunican et al. 2007).

While no studies have directly compared orlistat and sibutramine in adolescents, it appears that individuals taking sibutramine lose more weight than those on orlistat, but orlistat users have small reductions in blood pressure whereas sibutramine causes increases in blood pressure.

Concerns regarding adverse cardiovascular and psychological outcomes have limited the ability of the FDA to fully evaluate the safety of sibutramine for adolescents. Adverse GI effects are repeatedly reported for orlistat, but as with adults, this can be mediated by adjusting dietary fat intake. Metformin, a diabetic drug, has also been associated with weight loss in recent years. Only four small trials evaluating the efficacy of metformin for adolescents have been conducted so far; thus, further research is necessary before any recommendations can be made. Lifestyle modification (improved diet and increased physical activity) is key for any drug intervention to help (Dunican et al. 2007).

Adult Surgery

Adults who have a BMI > 40 kg/m^2 (or BMI > 35 with comorbid conditions) suffer from what is termed *extreme obesity* or *morbid obesity* and qualify for surgical treatment. Morbidly obese patients endure not only their excess weight but also a given number of other harmful conditions, including heart disease, sleep apnea, diabetes mellitus, hypertension, urinary incontinence, sexual hormone dysfunction, joint problems, and increased cancer incidence

(Latifi et al. 2002). Surgery can facilitate weight loss and improve the patient's comorbid conditions. While surgery offers potential health improvement to morbidly obese patients, the procedure involves significant risks. Before surgery can be considered as an option, patients must undergo treatment with medication and lifestyle interventions. Typically, patients who are at the highest risk for surgical mortality are the ones who would benefit most from having the surgery. Recently, concerns have been raised that patients are not well educated enough about potential adverse outcomes associated with treatment.

In 1991, the National Institutes of Health (NIH) issued bariatric surgery guidelines for severely obese adults who had tried, and failed at, nonsurgical approaches. Surgery for adult obesity has significantly increased since then. At the time of the original recommendations, no guidelines or recommendations were issued for children or adolescents. Since then, surgeons have performed and improved upon a number of weight-loss procedures, including the more popular Roux-en-Y gastric bypass and adjustable gastric banding procedures, which make the patient's stomach smaller (Steinbrook 2004). Currently, there are a number of surgical procedure options, including laparoscopic surgery. In laparoscopic surgery, a laparoscope, an instrument similar to a telescope that allows the physician to see inside the patient's abdomen, is inserted in the abdominal wall via a small incision (called a *laparoscopy*). The minimally invasive nature of laparoscopic surgery makes pain and recovery outcomes for the patient more favorable, but the risks and complications of surgical treatment still exist. Although surgery effects weight loss by reducing caloric intake, patients must change their lifestyle to achieve successful weight loss.

Gastric Bypass

First pioneered by Edward E. Mason and Chikashi Ito at the University of Iowa in the late 1960s, gastric bypass has become the most commonly performed bariatric surgery today due to its successful long-term weight-loss effects in morbidly obese patients. The procedure divides the patient's stomach into two parts, one significantly smaller than the other, in order to limit the amount of food a patient can take in. A stapling instrument is used to staple the smaller part, called the *proximal pouch*, separate from the larger part, called the *distal stomach*. Since food that enters the proximal pouch cannot later enter the distal stomach, we say that the distal stomach is bypassed. The food instead follows an alternative route that is constructed by the surgeon.

The surgeon connects the proximal pouch to the jejunum, which is the middle section of the small intestine. The small intestine is broken into three sections: the duodenum, the jejunum, and the ileum. Normally, food leaves the stomach and enters the duodenum first, then the jejunum and ileum, but since the proximal pouch is directly connected to the jejunum, the duodenum is bypassed, similarly to the distal stomach. The creation of a new opening, called the *stoma*, between the proximal pouch and the jejunum is referred to as a *gastrojejunostomy*. The portion of the jejunum through which food will move from the proximal pouch to the intestines is known as the Roux-en-Y limb due to the Y-shaped configuration formed. The procedure is thus commonly termed *Roux-en-Y gastric bypass*.

One particular subtype of bypass procedure, Dr. Mal Fobi's *Fobi pouch operation*, has gained notable attention in the 21st century due in part to Fobi's celebrity patients. The Fobi pouch operation, developed over the last two decades, includes smaller pouch and stoma sizes, a jejunal limb inserted between a cut edge of the proximal pouch and the distal pouch to address staple breakdown, the Silastic ring (a band used to reinforce the stoma), a gastrostomy (an opening in the stomach where a feeding tube can be inserted), and a marker for access to the stomach through the skin in addition to the original Roux-en-Y limb. While the operation appears to be effective for weight loss, a number of complications can occur. The most lethal postoperative complication, which can be indicated by tachycardia, is a leak from the stoma or proximal or distal pouches that goes unrecognized. Later complications that were sparsely seen in Fobi pouch patients were peptic ulcer disease, small bowel obstruction, ventral hernia, cholelithiasis, and psychiatric problems. Furthermore, weight-loss failure can still occur as a result of dilation of the stoma or pouches or disruption of the staple line (Fobi et al. 1998).

Celebrity Bypass Patients

Mal Fobi has been recognized for his modifications to gastric bypass due to his celebrity clientele who have gone public with their news of bypass surgery. The media attention given to stars who have received the Fobi pouch operation has led to a rise in the popularity of the surgical treatment of obesity.

The Fobi pouch operation in particular has been performed on a number of recognized names, including Randy Jackson and Etta James. The procedure can be distinguished from other bypass surgeries in three major ways: cutting the stomach instead of stapling, the band to prevent stomach widening, and the marker that identifies the stomach on an x-ray. These modifications are being adapted by a growing number of surgeons who perform gastric bypass, but Fobi remains the surgeon of the stars. Although the majority of Fobi's clientele is wealthy and Caucasian, African Americans and individuals of low socioeconomic status are more likely to be obese. Access to obesity surgery is limited by the high cost, ranging from $35,000 to $40,000, and varying health insurance coverage (Christian 2003).

Fobi's operative techniques have yielded positive outcomes for his famous patients, such as *American Idol* judge Randy Jackson. Jackson lost 100 lb. and 12 in. off his waist as a result of the surgery. Fobi performed Jackson's surgery laparoscopically, reducing his stomach size by 95 percent. Jackson elected to have the surgery as a last resort after trying a number of unsuccessful diets in order to improve his health and quality of life, which was marred by sleep apnea and type 2 diabetes. He has seen improvements in his comorbid conditions, but he has also had to limit his overall food intake and consumption of certain foods. As is the case for all gastric bypass patients, Jackson has said that bypass means lifelong changes for him, namely, exercise and limited food selection (Schneider et al. 2004).

Blues singer Etta James, the voice behind the well-known tune "At Last," became a patient of Fobi after hitting 400 lb. Fearful of having to leave the stage and even worried about dying, James sought the Fobi pouch operation for relief of her weight-related ill health. She was willing to risk the complications of surgery that Fobi emphasized for her age group (over 60) and, as a result, lost a significant amount of weight, weighing close to 220 lb. in 2003. As a result, James has seen an increase in her mobility, no longer needing a wheelchair, and has expanded her vocal range (Kinnon 2003).

While Randy Jackson and Etta James received the Fobi pouch technique for gastric bypass, other celebrities, including Star Jones, Carnie Wilson, and Al Roker, have undergone traditional Roux-en-Y gastric bypass surgery (Teeple 2008). All three stars have spoken out about the psychologic issues associated with their weight and gastric bypass. Jones has said she coped with her insecurities by splurging on unhealthy food items, seeing food as a source of comfort. She gained a large amount of weight in her early 40s until she became morbidly obese and underwent surgery at 307 lb. Despite the surgery-associated weight loss, Jones noted that her insecurities remained, and she began psychological therapy with a therapist who specialized in behavior modification for patients of weight-loss surgery (Reynolds 2007).

NBC news anchor Al Roker has expressed the value of such postoperative therapy to combat "emotional eating," which often led him to food for consolation. Roker has spoken out on his bypass and notes that the psychological issues motivating one to eat and gain weight in the first place cannot simply be erased by bypass surgery, which he received in 2001. Roker has used his journalism platform to interview adolescent patients who expressed similar emotional distress regarding the food restrictions imposed by bypass. As a result, some have come to view Roker as a spokesperson for bypass surgery. In response, Roker has spoken at length about the potential surgical complications, as much a reality as his surgical success. Roker conducted an NBC *Dateline* interview with Jennifer Butler, the widow of Mike Butler, in which she revealed how her husband lost his life to a postoperative stomal leak four days after his bypass surgery. During his subsequent hospitalization, he suffered from an infection and substantial internal bleeding and died a week later from pulmonary blood clots and a bleeding ulcer, according to doctors. Although the surgery cannot be blamed as the exact cause of Butler's death, the possibility remains that the mortal blood clots arose due to the leak-induced bed rest. Surgery can be imperative to redeem the health of morbidly obese patients, whose obese state may be more of a threat to their lives than the mortality risk of the operation itself. However, the average mortality risk remains significant; 1 in every 200 patients undergoing bypass dies (Roker 2004a, 2004b, 2004c).

The celebrity success stories can certainly provide inspiration for individuals considering weight-loss surgery as a last resort to combat their obesity. While their stories may give these individuals a figure to identify with, the public audience must realize that not everyone's surgical outcomes are the same. Any given person may have a negative experience with a procedure that yields positive outcomes for another individual and vice versa.

Other Procedures

In addition to gastric bypass, several other surgical procedures for the treatment of obesity exist. While bypass is recognized for significant weight loss and reversals in comorbidity, patients who receive bypass may be more prone to adverse postoperative symptoms and nutritional deficiencies (Steinbrook 2004). Vertical-banded gastroplasty (VBG), adjustable gastric banding, and biliopancreatic diversion are less commonly performed procedures that may result in less weight loss than gastric bypass. One procedure is not any more or less correct than another; rather, one may be more appropriate than another for a particular patient.

VBG restricts food intake similarly to gastric bypass by decreasing the stomach size (Latifi et al. 2002). Commonly called *stomach stapling*, VBG uses both staples and a band to create a smaller pouch near the gastroesophageal junction, where the esophagus and stomach meet. A very small outlet is created to allow food to flow from this pouch to the remainder of the stomach, where the food will be further digested and continue to move through the rest of the GI tract. Unlike gastric bypass, no portion of the GI tract is bypassed, or skipped. Thus, nutrients from the food are absorbed normally, but the rate at which food moves through the digestive system is slowed down. VBG is considered to be a restrictive approach, while bypass is considered to be both restrictive and malabsorptive.

VBG has become decreasingly common, in part due to the advent of adjustable gastric banding, introduced in 1983 (Latifi et al. 2002). The procedure is much like VBG, but the band used is adjustable and no stapling is involved. Adjustable gastric banding has the advantage of an adjustable band, and the procedure is reversible. Gastric banding uses a subcutaneous port, a point of access directly under the skin, that allows the surgeon to adjust the diameter of the outlet through which food leaves the small proximal pouch by injecting saline. This approach is restrictive and, unlike gastric bypass, does not affect nutrient absorption. Adjustable gastric banding is designed to cause long-term, gradual weight loss by reducing stomach capacity and forcing a change in patient eating habits to compensate. The band can be tightened or loosened by removing or injecting saline into the access port if circumstances, such as illness or pregnancy, demand a change in food intake. The LAP-BAND is the most popular of the adjustable gastric banding systems.

Laparoscopic adjustable gastric banding is considered an effective weight-loss option for morbid obesity that is minimally invasive and has a short recovery period. Patients typically see both a loss in weight and an improvement in or recovery from comorbid conditions as well as improvements in quality of life. Complications can still arise, necessitating reoperation. The most common is band slippage, which can result from too-loose band stitching on the anterior stomach wall or premature solid food intake.

While VBG and adjustable gastric banding both affect food intake and weight loss by restricting stomach size, biliopancreatic diversion takes a malabsorptive surgical approach similar to gastric bypass. During the procedure, the surgeon cuts and removes a portion of the stomach to decrease its size. The altered stomach is then connected to the ileum, the last section of the small intestine, allowing food to bypass the duodenum and the jejunum, the first two segments of the small intestine. As a result of the bypass of much of the small intestine, the risk of protein-calorie malnutrition and fat-soluble vitamin deficiency is rather high for biliopancreatic diversion patients relative to other procedures. Due to the complicated nature of the procedure and significant nutritional effects, biliopancreatic diversion is performed much less than the other procedures. A modified version of the procedure, biliopancreatic diversion with a duodenal switch, was developed to combat protein and fat-soluble vitamin malabsorption by incorporating a restrictive component (Zinzindohoue et al. 2003).

Adolescent Surgery

Although surgical treatment of obesity is increasingly common for adults, much debate remains over whether or not surgery should be recommended for obese adolescents. Some physicians argue that adolescent bariatric surgery is in fact safe and effective while others are still wary of potential complications and uncertain long-term outcomes. Reports of recent trends of bariatric surgery in the United States indicate that surgical incidence for young individuals has increased over time in spite of the lack of supportive evidence. Estimates in 2004 indicated that 500 children undergo surgery each year to control their weight, despite the controversy surrounding adolescent bariatric surgery (Roker 2004a).

In a study of 33 adolescents, 12 to 18 years of age, who met NIH criteria for severely obese adults (BMI $\geq$ 40 kg/m^2 or BMI $\geq$ 35 kg/m^2 with comorbid conditions, values that likely surpass the 85th and 95th percentile BMI pediatric cutoff points for being at risk for overweight and overweight) and who underwent surgery (largely gastric bypass, except for three gastroplasty patients), outcomes were generally positive (Sugerman et al. 2003). In addition to weight loss, the adolescents experienced improvement or resolution of comorbid conditions, including sleep apnea, type 2 diabetes mellitus, degenerative joint disease, gastroesophageal reflux symptoms, pseudotumor cerebri, systemic hypertension, and polycystic ovary syndrome. Most patients had three or more preoperative comorbid conditions. Significant weight loss was seen at 1, 5, 10, and 14 years postoperation, except for five patients who regained the weight 5–10 years after surgery. All of the adolescents reported improvements in self-image and social interaction within one year of surgery. There were two deaths among the group, one at two years and one at six years postoperatively, but they were likely not linked to the surgery itself. Overall, results mirror those seen in adults who suffered similar comorbid conditions. It remains to be determined what the optimal timing of the surgery and procedure is. In addition, there is little data on quality of life changes or long-term outcomes. Preventive measures are still critical and necessary to combat overweight in adolescence.

The majority of adolescent obesity surgery patients are female, Caucasian, and ages 15–19 and have private insurance, have no comorbid conditions, and opt for gastric bypass (Tsai et al. 2007). The majority of hospitals that perform adolescent bariatric surgery performed the procedure on only a few adolescents per year. Some have suggested that specialized centers for adolescent bariatric surgery are needed, while others argue that given the low volume of procedures done, the best approach is to perform the adolescent surgery at a high-volume adult center with pediatric surgeons involved. Specified adolescent centers may provide more specialized postoperative support, such as psychological and metabolic support, that adult centers may not offer. A 2004 consensus report on adolescent bariatric surgery created guidelines for the selection of candidates for the surgical treatment of adolescent overweight and recommended the development of centers specializing in adolescent bariatric care (Schilling et al. 2008). As of 2003, most adolescent procedures took place at hospitals that had a high volume of obesity surgery procedures (over 200 per year). The rate of complications is higher at low-volume compared to high-volume centers (Weller and Hannan 2006).

Use of surgical treatment for adolescent overweight is gaining popularity in the 21st century but is still uncommon relative to adult surgical treatment. A lack of data on long-term outcomes prevents physicians and researchers from recommending surgery because of a lack of information on safety and efficacy for adolescents. Concerns also exist regarding the need for specialized psychological postoperative care in adolescents as well as the unanswered questions about how surgery at a young age affects future growth and development.

Surgical Outcomes and Complications

Surgical complications can be categorized according to the time at which they occur relative to the operation itself. *Perioperative* refers to complications that occur during the surgery, *postoperative* refers to complications that occur after the procedure, and *late* refers to complications that develop over time. While perioperative complications can be avoided by careful planning and surgeon execution, nonspecific complications can arise at any time, whether they involve an unexpected bad reaction to a medication or anesthesia-related injuries. One of the most lethal complications, a leak from the anastomosis (the opening created by the gastrojejunostomy) or proximal or distal gastric pouches, occurs postoperatively and may result in death if not treated immediately. Unfortunately, a leak is not always easy to detect without external symptoms, but tachycardia, a rapid pulse, is typically indicative of leakage in gastric bypass patients (Fobi et al. 1998). Other postoperative complications include deep vein thrombosis, pulmonary embolus, stomal ulcers and stomal stenosis, or narrowing of the stoma. Early ambulation, which refers to the act of moving about, is recommended for patients to avoid and/or reduce the presence of such complications.

Nutritional and vitamin deficiencies are perhaps the most prominent yet treatable complications that persist late after surgery. These include but are not limited to protein-calorie malnutrition and vitamin B_{12}, iron, magnesium, and calcium deficiencies. Fat-soluble vitamins A, D, and E may leave the body more readily and escape absorption, particularly in bypass patients (Fobi et al. 1998). Patients can compensate for nutrient loss with routine intake of oral supplements. Deficiencies commonly result from malabsorptive rather than restrictive procedures, but any patient who undergoes gastric surgery may be faced with nutritional complications. Patients must follow a balanced diet while consuming a smaller amount of food.

Several surgical complications have been documented for gastric bypass patients, perhaps as a result of the procedure's popularity. A commonly recurring and unique complication in bypass patients is *dumping syndrome*. Dumping syndrome, also known as rapid gastric emptying, refers to the symptoms, such as nausea and cramps, that result when undigested food moves or is "dumped" from the stomach to the small intestine too quickly.

VBG patients often experience gastroesophageal reflux. VBG has fewer maladaptive nutrient effects than bypass but is less popular. Pros and cons can thus be named for each respective operation, and technical complications, whether a leak or a tear within the surgical area, can likely result from each.

Surgery has the potential for substantial weight loss of more than half the initial excess weight in the first one to two years. Ideally, weight loss stabilizes later on, given that dietary and other lifestyle interventions are maintained. Equally important, a number of conditions can be improved or eliminated, including type 2 diabetes and hypertension (eliminated for two-thirds to three-fourths of patients); patients may also experience alleviated sleep apnea, ameliorated hypoventilation, improved lipid profiles, decreased cytokine levels, corrected sex hormone abnormalities, alleviated urinary incontinence and joint pain, and improved quality of life and psychological outlook. While the change in physical appearance that comes with weight loss is meaningful for many patients, the improvement in health status is the critical outcome that physicians strive for in order to extend the life span.

Unfortunately, surgery sometimes fails to deliver substantial weight loss, and patients can require a reversal of the procedure and/or reoperation. The qualification for failed outcomes is less than 40 percent loss of excess weight (Latifi et al. 2002). Even patients who do lose enough weight may gain back the lost weight, likelier due to continuous snacking on foods with high caloric density or lack of exercise than due to stoma or pouch expansion. Reoperation for gastric surgery runs a higher risk of mortality, morbidity, and complications as compared to the primary surgery. In addition to weight-loss failure, unresolved comorbid conditions can qualify a patient for operative conversion to another gastric technique, for example, partial biliopancreatic diversion.

The aforementioned procedures (VBG, gastric bypass, and adjustable gastric band) can be performed laparoscopically. Laparoscopic has advantages over open surgery, including a shorter recovery, less-invasive nature, and reduced chance of hernia. Since adjustable gastric banding is a newer surgery, uncertainty remains over the long-term safety and efficacy of the laparoscopic procedure. Results of the laparoscopic gastric bypass and open technique appear to be comparable and, interestingly enough, the laparoscopic version takes longer.

The success of weight-loss strategies is limited. Results from the NWCR do provide some hope that weight loss can be achieved and maintained in the long term. The key to slowing or stopping the obesity epidemic may be to prevent obesity in the first place. We have discussed obesogenic social and physical environments, including schools and neighborhoods, and the efforts on the part of employers to promote health among their employees. Some weight-loss drugs are currently approved for use in obese adults, but there are potentially harmful side effects. Surgical procedures for weight loss, although not without risk, can be successful and improve the health status of patients who undergo these procedures, especially if patients also change their lifestyles.

6

Economic Costs of Obesity

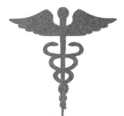

The economic consequences of obesity are sobering. The costs associated with obesity add even more strain to the already overburdened health care budgets and financially stretched public health systems of countries, including the United States. When creating a budget for health care, financial planners must have an estimate of what the costs will be so that money can be directed to the greatest health priorities. Everyone is angling for their piece of the pie, so to speak. Money is needed for obesity prevention programs, and money is needed to treat the health-related consequences of obesity, such as type 2 diabetes. Obesity is a threat to the current and future economic viability of many countries because it pulls resources away from investment in technology and other areas of the economy and limits productivity. If obesity could have been prevented, it is estimated that the United States could have saved about $45.8 billion in 1990, which would have amounted to 6.8 percent of total health care expenditures for that year (Wolf and Colditz 1994). In 2001 the total economic costs of obesity in the United States were estimated at $117 billion. By 2030, overweight and obesity could cost as much as $957 billion, which breaks down to $1 out of every $6 spent on health care and would be as much as 18 percent of total health care costs (Y. Wang et al. 2008). These cost projections are likely to be significant underestimations because of the increase in the prevalence of obesity and the fact that per capita health care costs for obesity-related diseases are rising faster than per capita total health care costs.

In this chapter, we will discuss the economic costs of obesity broken down by type of cost.

DIRECT COSTS

Direct costs relate specifically to the cost of preventing, diagnosing, or treating obesity or obesity-related conditions, like coronary heart disease (CHD). Estimates of these costs usually take into account expenses incurred from visits to doctors' offices, hospitalizations, nursing home care, treatment, and medications.

Expenditures on obesity in 1995 were estimated at $51.6 billion for chronic obesity-related diseases, or 5.7 percent of U.S. health care expenditures (Wolf and Colditz 1998). In 2003, direct costs associated with obesity were estimated at $75 billion (Finkelstein 2004).

The following five obesity-associated diseases account for 85 percent of the health care expenditures on obesity: hypertension, hyperlipidemia, type 2 diabetes, coronary artery disease, and stroke. Almost 60 percent of the cost of type 2 diabetes in 1990 was for obesity-related type 2 diabetes. The direct cost of obesity-related cardiovascular disease in 1990 was estimated to be $28 billion (Wolf and Colditz 1994). The rising prevalence of obesity combined with the growing list of obesity-related diseases has led to the expectation that direct costs will rise precipitously.

The annual medical expenditures for obese individuals are 37 percent higher than expenditures for normal-weight individuals. Between 1987 and 2001, total U.S. medical expenditures attributable to the rising prevalence of obesity rose by 12 percent as compared to spending on normal-weight people (Thorpe et al. 2004). Obesity-related medical expenditures, which are about 9.1 percent by some estimates, now rival medical expenditures related to smoking in the United States, which are between 6.5 and 14.5 percent of total annual U.S. health care costs, depending on the data source.

As compared to normal-weight individuals, obese people utilize more health care resources, are hospitalized more often, and use more medications. One study showed that compared to people with a body mass index (BMI) < 25, people with a BMI of 30 to 34.9 utilized 17 percent more outpatient services and 34 percent more inpatient services. Average health care costs also vary by the degree of obesity. Even overweight, moderately obese, and severely obese individuals impose different costs on the health care system. Several

Table 6.1
Weight Classifications by Body Mass Index (BMI)

Weight Classification	BMI
Normal weight	18.5–24.9
Overweight	25.0–29.9
Obese	30.0–34.9
Severely obese	35.0–39.9
Extremely obese	>40.0

studies have demonstrated that average health care costs for the obese (BMI ≥ 30) and overweight (BMI 25 to 29.9) are higher than for normal-weight individuals (BMI 18.5 to 24.9). Compared to a normal-weight group, the average health care cost for the obese was over $1,000 higher, and the cost for overweight was higher by $340 for the year 2001 (Thorpe et al. 2004). Annual health care costs in 2002 among the severely obese (BMI 35 to 39.9) were 50 percent higher than normal-weight individuals. And extremely obese (BMI ≥ 40) individuals had double the annual health care costs, a 100 percent increase, as compared to their normal-weight counterparts (Andreyeva et al. 2004).

Over the course of a year, the health care costs for overweight individuals (BMI ≥ 27.9) are higher than for normal-weight individuals, mainly because of prescription drugs. Not only do obese individuals have higher medical costs due to more hospitalizations and outpatient visits, but also they use more prescription drugs than nonobese individuals. Specifically, obese individuals use more antidiabetic agents, heart medication, pain relievers, and asthma medication (Raebel et al. 2004). Obese people (BMI ≥ 30) have more visits to their primary care doctor, visit more specialty care clinics, and have more diagnostic tests as compared to nonobese (BMI < 30) individuals. Obese people have greater total medical charges as compared to nonobese individuals (Bertakis and Azari 2005). In summary, the chronic diseases from which obese people suffer cost more to treat due to higher use of medical care, specifically greater use of prescription medication.

Lifetime Medical Costs

How do overweight and obesity impact lifetime medical costs? One study examined lifetime medical costs that can be attributed to overweight and obesity and found that costs varied by age and race. The results showed that being overweight did not result in any extra lifetime medical costs, except among white women. Twenty-year-old overweight white women can expect lifetime medical costs to be about $8,120. Sixty-five-year-old overweight white women can expect lifetime medical costs to be about $4,560. There are also excess lifetime costs associated with being obese. The lifetime costs for 20-year-old obese black women were the lowest at $5,340 and highest for white women at $21,550. Starting at age 65, lifetime costs attributable to obesity were highest among obese black men ($19,270) and lowest among obese black women ($4,660). The lifetime costs for 20-year-old very obese (BMI $\geq$ 35) adults ranged from $14,580 for black men to $29,460 for white women. The lifetime costs for 65-year-old very obese adults ranged from $7,590 for black women to $25,300 for white women (Finkelstein et al. 2008). In young adulthood, the lifetime medical costs related to obesity are slightly higher than the lifetime medical costs of a normal-weight person. However, as they age, the costs for an obese person become greater as compared to a normal-weight person. The results of this study also show that the lifetime cost of obesity starting when a person turns 65 is much higher than for a normal-weight person. This places an enormous financial burden on the Medicare system in the United States. Another study confirmed the findings for the over-65 age group (Yang and Hall 2008). This study followed about 28,000 men and women starting at age 65. The elderly men and women who were overweight or obese had, respectively, 6 to 13 percent and 11 to 17 percent more lifetime health care expenditures as compared with their normal-weight peers. These estimates included inpatient, outpatient, prescription drug, and nursing home costs. The lifetime health costs for men and women who were obese at age 65 were estimated to be, respectively, $190,657 and $223,629. On average, the extra health care costs for each overweight individual were estimated at $15,000 and for each obese individual about $26,000. On a population level, the researchers estimate that this could translate to $400 billion in extra health care expenditures for overweight and obesity among the elderly (Yang and Hall 2008).

Lifetime Costs of Obesity-Related Diseases

The lifetime costs of treating hypertension, hypercholesterolemia, type 2 diabetes, CHD, and stroke all increase with increasing BMI, according to a study of adults aged 35 to 64. The researchers in this study categorized people as nonobese (BMI 22.5–27.4), mildly obese (BMI 27.5–32.4), moderately obese (BMI 32.5-37.4), and severely obese (BMI $\geq$ 37.5). The cost of treating all five conditions in a nonobese 45- to 54-year-old man is $19,600 and increases to $24,000 for the mildly obese, $29,600 for the moderately obese, and $36,500 for the severely obese. The cost of treating these obesity-related diseases among women aged 45 to 54 years was higher: $18,800 for the nonobese, $23,200 for the mildly obese, $28,700 for the moderately obese, and $35,300 for the severely obese. In men and women combined, CHD is estimated to account for half of all lifetime medical costs. When the researchers looked at women separately, type 2 diabetes accounted for the greatest lifetime cost for those who were categorized as mildly, moderately, or severely obese (Thompson 1999).

Some researchers have theorized that premature death, especially among the severely obese, may actually result in lower lifetime health care costs. That is, obese people die at a younger age due to the high prevalence of chronic diseases. As a result, they do not utilize as much health care as their nonobese counterparts. However, closer examination of the data does not support this theory. After accounting for the difference in survival between obese and normal-weight individuals, one study showed that the lifetime medical costs for the obese are not lower. Early death due to obesity does not offset the medical costs incurred by the obese. In fact, the lifetime medical costs are higher among the obese and increase with increasing BMI regardless of race or gender (Finkelstein et al. 2008). As mentioned earlier in this chapter, the same study found that lifetime medical costs were not increased for the overweight, with the exception of white women.

Children

There is not much information regarding the economic burden of obesity in children, but one study examined changes in the number of diagnoses of obesity-attributable diseases over time and calculated the annual hospital costs associated with these diagnoses. Using the National Hospital Discharge Survey, researchers found that between two time periods, 1979–1981 and 1997–1999, the percentage of children aged 6 to 17 years old discharged with a diagnosis of diabetes nearly doubled, obesity and gallbladder disease tripled, and sleep apnea increased fivefold (Wang and Dietz 2002).

The rise in obesity-associated diseases resulted in increasingly longer average hospital stays for children over the last 20 years, and longer hospital stays mean higher hospital bills. The hospital costs associated with the increases in obesity-related diseases among children were estimated at $35 million annually in the years 1979–1981 and $127 million in 1997–1999. This represents a threefold increase in hospital costs over two decades (Wang and Dietz 2002).

How does overweight and obesity in young adulthood and middle age relate to Medicare expenditures in older age (≥65 years)? Not surprisingly, being overweight or obese in young adulthood or middle age resulted in higher total average annual Medicare charges. The annual charge for women who were obese in young adulthood and middle age was $9,612 as compared to $6,224 for women who were of normal weight. The annual charge for a man who was obese in young adulthood and middle age was $10,128 as compared to $7,205 for normal-weight men (Daviglus et al. 2004). The results of this study highlight the potential for the aging obese population of the United States to impose enormous costs on the Medicare system.

It is estimated that future direct costs to the U.S. health care system will double every decade.

INDIRECT COSTS

Indirect costs are the decreases in economic activity that are associated with diseases or early death that can be blamed on obesity. Obesity may increase indirect costs by decreasing productivity because people cannot work due to obesity-related disease. Estimation of the indirect costs of obesity may take into account the value of income lost from variables such as sick days, restriction of activities, decreased efficiency in performing a task, early retirement, disability pensions, lower wages, and future earnings lost by premature death from obesity.

In 1995, the indirect costs of obesity were estimated at $47.6 billion. In 2000, the indirect costs of obesity to the United States were estimated at $56 billion (Wolf and Colditz 1998). The indirect costs associated with obesity are estimated to be much larger than the direct costs. Higher BMI is related to increases in sick days and short-term disability and higher health care costs (Burton 1998). Very obese men and women with obesity-related chronic diseases were estimated to miss work, respectively, 4 days/year and 5.5 days/year.

Obesity has a serious detrimental effect on individual earnings. It has been demonstrated that obese people have more trouble finding and retaining jobs and that obesity is associated with diminished earnings and lower wages (Cawley 2004). Employers have to pay higher health insurance premiums for obese employees, and they incur the costs of absenteeism and decreased productivity. In 1998, obesity-related absenteeism cost U.S. employers an estimated $2.4 billion (Thompson et al. 1998). In 1998, it was estimated that obesity resulted in 39.2 million days of lost work, 239 million restricted-activity days, and 89.5 million bed days per year (Wolf and Colditz 1998). Complications from obesity contribute to indirect costs. Because a large portion of obesity-related premature death is from CHD, it is estimated to account for 48 percent of the total indirect costs of obesity. Non–insulin-dependent diabetes accounts for 17.5 percent and osteoarthritis for 17.1 percent. Osteoarthritis resulted in a large proportion of total indirect costs of obesity because many people with this condition have restricted activity at work, take sick days, or have bed days (Colditz 1999).

Limitations of Calculations of Economic Costs of Obesity

The economic costs of overweight and obesity are not easy to estimate. The estimates and projections of the economic costs of obesity certainly all underestimate the true costs to society. Researchers are now arguing for a standardized method of calculating the costs associated with obesity. Standardization allows for comparisons to be made across studies. For example, everyone should agree to use the same BMI cutoff points to define obesity. It is difficult to compare costs across studies when they define obesity in different ways. For example, one study may have defined obesity as BMI $\geq$ 30, while another study defined it as BMI $\geq$ 27.9. There should also be a standardized list of obesity-related diseases to include in cost estimates. Otherwise, when policy makers try to make decisions about how to allocate funds for obesity, they are comparing apples to oranges.

There is a need for more data sets that have reliable BMI information and accurate numbers on diseases associated with obesity, especially among minority populations. It is important to know the burden imposed by obesity-related diseases in different ethnic groups so that costs of treating these illnesses can be accurately estimated. As we noted earlier, the prevalence of obesity-related diseases varies across racial and ethnic groups, so knowing the full economic cost hinges on knowing the extent of disease.

The risk for certain diseases increases starting at a BMI of 25. Most calculations of cost do not include people who are classified as overweight (BMI 25–29.9), instead focusing on the obese (BMI $\geq$ 30). The exclusion of those classified as overweight in estimations of the costs of obesity means we are not getting a full picture of the substantial costs, direct and indirect, associated with the health effects of being overweight.

What conditions and illnesses should be included in calculations of the costs of obesity? For example, sleep apnea is not included in cost estimates, nor are all cancers. Some studies include the cost of treating mental disorders or respiratory conditions, and others do not. In addition to the cancers we know are associated with obesity (esophagus, pancreas, colon and rectum, female breast [postmenopausal], endometrium, and kidney [renal cell]) but that haven't been included in estimates, there are other cancers for which evidence suggests obesity is a contributing factor. As more evidence on the relation between obesity and these cancers emerges, cost estimates may need to be correspondingly updated. The estimation of the costs associated with obesity will have to be flexible enough to accommodate evolving scientific evidence linking obesity to a longer and longer list of diseases and disorders.

Other challenges in estimating cost arise in deciding what data to use. Some researchers may have used data that included expenses related to hospitalizations, outpatient care, and physicians visits but that excluded cost information on nursing homes or claims for medical equipment. Sometimes the data are not available for all the different areas of cost. This is yet another reason researchers argue that an effort needs to be made to standardize the list of costs included in economic calculations and why the estimates we do have may underestimate the true costs of obesity.

Another problem in analyzing the data on obesity is that many health care payers do not provide coverage for the treatment of obesity. For example, in the National Hospital Discharge Survey study mentioned earlier in the chapter, physicians may not diagnose obesity in children as a primary illness even if it is clearly the diagnosis because insurance companies may not pay for hospital stays related to obesity. Instead, they may diagnose diabetes or sleep apnea as the primary illness, which results in an underestimation of costs associated with obesity.

Weight Gain

Cost estimates do not take into account the impact of weight gain over the life span on increasing costs. And there is limited research available relating weight gain to health care costs. One study in female nurses did calculate the direct costs associated with weight gain in relation to type 2 diabetes and CHD. The direct costs of type 2 diabetes attributable to adult weight gain of 5–10 kg, 11–19.9 kg, or ≥20 kg were $1.56 billion, $4.61 billion, and $6.88 billion in 1993 dollars, respectively. The direct costs of CHD attributable to adult weight gain of 5–10 kg, 11–19.9 kg, or ≥20 kg were $2.99 billion, $4.76 billion, and $4.2 billion in 1993 dollars, respectively. Weight gain increases not only the risk of developing type 2 diabetes and CHD (as discussed in Chapter 5) but also the costs associated with these illnesses (Wolf and Colditz 1996). Given the increases in health care costs since 1993, these numbers likely significantly underestimate the current costs of weight gain.

As discussed in Chapter 5, overweight and obesity greatly impact quality of life, and to assign a dollar value to someone's decrease in quality of life is impossible. There are also social and personal costs incurred by individuals that are not accounted for in calculations of the total cost of obesity. For example, the weight-loss industry is a big business. And it is estimated that

Americans spend $40 billion a year on weight-loss programs, books, and products.

Relationship of Poverty and Obesity

Obesity and poverty are inversely related to one another. That is, higher rates of obesity correlate with lower levels of socioeconomic status. Why does this relationship exist? The obesity-poverty relationship is a self-perpetuating cycle. Obesity limits economic opportunities, and in turn poverty increases the chances of becoming obese (Runge 2007). Obesity, as we discussed in Chapter 5, is related to a number of chronic diseases and in many cases decreases physical functioning. Obese people are often unable to work because they are ill and cannot physically do a job; then, their wages decrease or they lose their jobs. Unfortunately, the burden of obesity is often felt by those who are the least able to afford it. For example, an obese person who is ill with a chronic disease such as diabetes often cannot afford and/or does not have access to health care. The lost wages and cost of health care often plunge economically compromised households into further poverty.

Being overweight in adolescence or young adulthood has important economic implications later in life. One study followed over 10,000 overweight adolescents and young adults for eight years and found that both men and women married less frequently than those who had not been overweight. Women had lower household incomes and higher rates of household poverty as compared to women who had not been overweight adolescents and young adults (Gortmaker et al. 1993). Discrimination against overweight or obese individuals cannot be discounted as a contributor to the obesity-poverty relationship.

How does poverty increase the chances of becoming obese? It would be natural to assume that when a household has a limited budget for food, that members would consume fewer calories, right? Well, it turns out that this assumption is wrong. When people have to limit their spending on food, they choose cheaper foods, which happen to be the more energy-dense variety and contain more sugars, fats, and carbohydrates. Purchasing fruits and vegetables, lean meats, or fish is just not cost-effective for low-income households (Drewnowski and Darmon 2005). People who are poor tend to live in low-income neighborhoods, which increases their risk of obesity even further, as we discussed previously.

Cost-Effectiveness of Treatments

When health care groups, insurers, researchers, doctors, and politicians who lobby for how to allocate money in the health care system make spending decisions, they want to know that the money for obesity will go toward programs that have been demonstrated to be effective. Otherwise, spending the money on unproven programs is a waste of taxpayer or company dollars. Cost-effectiveness relates the cost of an intervention (usually in terms of money) relative to achieving a certain outcome. One metric might be "this program costs $X for each pound of weight lost" in a particular intervention.

Some have argued that estimating the cost-effectiveness of prevention and treatment is more important than estimating the costs of obesity to society. They argue that the numbers that really matter are the ones telling us what interventions are working to prevent obesity and bring about weight loss that is maintained over the long term.

Unfortunately, there is not much information on the long-term effectiveness of interventions to combat obesity. Many of the interventions and programs mentioned in Chapter 5 have never been evaluated for cost-effectiveness. The information we do have indicates that the cost-effectiveness of many treatments for obesity is not encouraging. For example, the cost-effectiveness of dietary counseling, behavior therapy, and surgery for weight loss is low. An economic evaluation of different types of weight-loss interventions in overweight and obese women found that interventions that combine diet, exercise, and behavior modification were not only more effective but also more cost-effective than interventions that focused on diet only, diet and prescription drugs (e.g., orlistat), or diet and exercise (Roux et al. 2006). The three-component intervention costs $12,600 per quality-adjusted life year (QALY) gained, compared with no intervention. QALY is a measure of health during a year of life and ranges from 0 to 1. Researchers assign a QALY to someone based on his or her health status information. A QALY of 1 is assigned to someone who has a year of perfect health. If someone is ill, that person may get a QALY of 0.6 or 0.5, and so forth, depending on his or her state of health. One drawback of Roux and colleagues' analysis is that it took into consideration an intervention period of only six months and a six-month maintenance period. Is six months a long enough period of time in which to effect behavior change that will last? Following the women for longer than six months after the intervention may have answered the question of whether the women in the diet, exercise, and behavior modification group were able to keep the weight off. It would be interesting to know which intervention provided the best value over the long term.

In 2006, the American Dietetic Association (ADA) published a review of the existing literature on interventions for pediatric obesity. The position of the ADA is that family-based (for kids from age 5 to 12 years) and school-based (for adolescents) multicomponent interventions offer the most benefit.

Multicomponent interventions include behavioral counseling, promotion of physical activity, parent training and modeling, dietary counseling, and nutrition education. The ADA also recommends community-based and environmental interventions, although there is not yet enough evidence to state whether these types of interventions are truly effective (ADA 2006).

Planet Health, the school-based intervention we described in Chapter 5, is an example of a cost-effective intervention. Remember, the goal of Planet Health is to reduce obesity in middle school children through lessons designed to lower TV viewing, decrease consumption of high-fat foods, increase fruit and vegetable intake, and increase moderate and vigorous physical activity. The estimated costs of implementing the Planet Health program include the cost of training teachers, Planet Health curriculum book, salaries for the Planet Health trainer and an assistant, cost of food during teacher training, and $400–$600 per school as an incentive to participate in Planet Health. Planet Health cost $14 per student per year to run in the intervention schools. The program is estimated to prevent about 6 out of 310 female students in the intervention schools from becoming overweight adults. The researchers also estimated how much money could be saved in the future by preventing the girls from becoming overweight adults. The program could save $15,887 in direct costs (health care) and $25,104 in indirect costs (lost productivity) and would result in a cost of $4,305 per QALY saved, which is cost-effective (Wang et al. 2003). Planet Health is a great example of how investing in interventions may have up-front costs, but if the intervention is effective and cost-effective, it will result in lower future health care costs.

Cost Associated with Abdominal Obesity

In Chapter 4, we discussed the health risks associated with the distribution of body fat, in particular those associated with abdominal adiposity. The estimations of the direct cost of obesity on the health care system have all been based on studies using BMI. Economists and health researchers are constantly working to improve estimates of the cost of obesity to society and the health care system. As noted in Chapter 2, BMI is not an ideal way to measure obesity because it is not a direct measure of body fatness. One ongoing study endeavors to determine how abdominal obesity impacts health care costs. The Prospective Obesity Cohort of Economic Evaluation and Determinants (PROCEED) is an Internet-based study of adults in the United States, Canada, the United Kingdom, and Germany. Recruitment for U.S. participants took place via e-mail invitation in 2004. The goal of the study is to compare the use of health care services among normal-weight (BMI 20–24), overweight (BMI

25–29.9), and obese (BMI $\geq$ 30) participants who may or may not have abdominal adiposity. Abdominal adiposity is defined as having a waist circumference of greater than 40 inches in men and greater than 35 inches in women. Each participant received a scale and a tape measure with which to report his or her weight and waist circumference, respectively. A small preliminary study published in 2008 estimated the costs associated with abdominal obesity among U.S. participants over a three-month period. There were 100 normal-weight, 474 overweight, and 493 obese participants. Overweight participants who had abdominal obesity were found to use more prescriptions for diabetes, depression, and insomnia as compared to overweight participants without abdominal obesity. Preliminary analyses revealed that abdominal obesity may be a better predictor of health care costs among the overweight and not obese people (Wolf et al. 2008). The publication of more results from the PRO-CEED study in the coming years should help further the understanding of how abdominal obesity influences health care costs.

SUMMARY

Employers, taxpayers, private insurers, and poor people will bear the cost of the obesity epidemic. The medical consequences of the obesity epidemic are staggering in terms of cost. In this chapter, the direct costs of obesity were discussed in terms of lifetime medical costs and the lifetime costs of treating obesity-related diseases. In addition, we discussed how complications from overweight and obesity impact indirect costs such as obesity-related absenteeism. And we touched upon the hurdles faced by researchers trying to accurately estimate the economic costs of obesity. Last, we highlighted a few studies that are investigating the cost-effectiveness of select interventions.

7

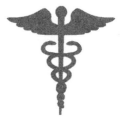

What's Next?

We've spent a lot of time talking about the consequences of obesity and the small to modest successes in the prevention and treatment of obesity. It is worthwhile now to look at the future and what leading scientists see as the future. Dr. Marion Nestle, a leading food researcher, offers a bit of simple advice:

> Eat less (starting with sugary drinks) and move more. Understand how food marketers manipulate consumer behavior. Be citizens, not consumers!
> (Nestle, personal communication)

NOVEL INTERVENTIONS

On the research front, interventions are also taking a new look at obesity. Let's look at one particularly promising example. Be Fit, Be Well is a weight-loss and maintenance study funded by the National Heart, Lung, and Blood Institute. This study further addresses one of the issues we've discussed in earlier chapters—the disproportionate burden of obesity in lower-income and racial and ethnic minority populations—by delivering the intervention through community health centers. Community health centers provide primary medical care to neighborhood residents who are uninsured or have limited insurance coverage. The Be Fit, Be Well intervention is delivered in a network of Boston-area health centers that serve a low-income and racially and ethnically diverse population.

Be Fit, Be Well marks a shift from previous interventions that focused on explicit calorie restriction by instead focusing intervention messages on lifestyle changes and goal setting for behavior change. The intervention also takes advantages of health technology such as Internet messages, tailored print materials, phone contact, and pedometers for tracking physical activity. Finally, the intervention considers the social and physical environment in which participants live.

So what does the Be Fit, Be Well intervention entail? It is a two-year intervention that compares electronic support (through the Web or a combination of tailored print and interactive, computerized telephone messages) to usual care plus an untailored weight-loss booklet. The intervention has a third arm, discussed in more detail below, which comprises electronic support plus personal support. The intervention has strong ties to the primary care setting where it is delivered. The intervention itself focuses on three features.

First, the intervention goals are tailored to the individual's needs. The goals, detailed below, include things like portion control, goal setting, managing barriers to behavior change, preventing relapse, healthy shopping, and label reading. The goals are designed to produce an energy deficit (fewer calories in than out) and to be concrete, readily achievable, easily self-monitored, and capable of being easily integrated into one's daily activities. Because nuanced phrasing of goals can be confusing and inhibit their adoption, the goals are designed to be concrete, however they are delivered. Goals are also presented with additional information to contextualize the recommendation and help participants feel that the intervention understands the context in which they live. For example, the intervention tells participants that they should not eat fast food but also provides a list of foods that participants should try if they absolutely must visit a fast food restaurant.

The intervention also provides training in the skills necessary to achieve and maintain weight loss. The skills training materials present instruction in behavior change strategies to achieve the intervention goals and introduce additional weight-loss and hypertension management goals. For example, when the recommendation to consume at least six servings of whole grains is given, the intervention materials also include information about where such foods can be purchased (given that there is only one full-service supermarket within easy reach of the participants), how to identify whole-grain products, how to integrate whole grains into one's daily diet (given that very few study participants have eaten such products), and alternatives if whole grains are not available.

Self-management of weight loss is the key to Be Fit, Be Well's plan for long-term successful weight loss and maintenance of that weight loss. Self-management is achieved through several intervention features. Tailoring makes printed materials relevant to an individual and includes features that are friendly to low-literacy populations such as short, simple text and lots of graphic images. To make the materials engaging and interesting, they also include stories and testimonials, games, and question and answer sections.

Be Fit, Be Well also asks participants to develop their own action plans, so they choose which behaviors to change and what the goal for that change will be. Participants select three goals to work on over the course of the intervention from a list of diet and physical activity goal options. All participants are also asked to have a goal for adherence to their hypertension medication regimen as all participants in the study suffer from high blood pressure. Every 12 weeks, participants are given the option of changing their diet and physical activity goals. Participants then self-monitor their adherence to their selected goals. The study checks in with participants every week (via phone or the Internet) to record their self-monitoring data, provide tailored feedback based on progress, and review the behavioral skills lessons for the week.

At baseline, all participants are given a goal of 10,000 steps per day and consuming no sugar-sweetened beverages. This goal is delivered as a prescription from the participants' primary care provider, integrating the Be Fit, Be Well study into the primary care delivered through the community health center. It also reinforces to the participants the importance of the behavior change in the eyes of their physician. Physician recommendation for behavior change is another aspect of weight-loss success as behavior change messages delivered by physicians are often viewed as having greater authority than generic messages such as those delivered through mass media.

The goals in the intervention allow for the final key feature, namely, self-monitoring of behaviors to track changes. In order to achieve an energy deficit and, thus, weight loss, participants must change behavior and maintain that change.

The intervention seeks to address several issues that previous interventions have not: It is specifically focused on weight loss in African Americans, who have typically seen less success than whites in weight-loss trials. Be Fit, Be Well also looks ahead at how the intervention might be disseminated if it proves successful. As community health centers are a resource of primary care across the nation, the approach used in Be Fit, Be Well can easily be adapted to other communities. In thinking about how to best serve African Americans, the Be Fit, Be Well investigators determined that previous studies may have had limited success because they failed to address the cultural and community needs of the study participants. Be Fit, Be Well tests whether providing in-person social environmental support through group support sessions, community walking groups, coaching by a community health worker, and information on community resources and access will enhance the effectiveness of the intervention. Individuals in this intervention arm receive phone calls from a community health worker 18 times over the course of the intervention, participate in 12 biweekly support group sessions, and receive information on using community resources and how to navigate the physical and social environment in which they live. Group sessions include walking groups led by a community health worker that aim to facilitate social support and training in the skill (walking for exercise) target. Walking outings may also be linked to other skills such as a walk to the grocery store to read labels or to a fast food establishment to talk about healthier menu items. Phone calls delivered by a community health worker aim to enhance and sustain motivation in participants by providing additional coaching. The calls review self-monitoring goals, identify barriers to success and potential responses to those barriers, establish new goals, and discuss how to use community resources to help achieve goals. Finally, this arm provides information on the community's environment and how it can help with reaching goals. For example, participants receive a list of interesting walking destinations (parks, stores, public transportation stops) along with the number of steps to reach each destination. Be Fit, Be Well also has an eye to the cost issues we discussed in Chapter 6 and will evaluate the cost-effectiveness of this additional intervention component.

The specific goals of the Be Fit, Be Well intervention are as follows:

Diet Goals
1. Eliminate consumption of sugar-sweetened beverages. Choose from alternatives including
   a. Water
   b. Flavored water (carbonated and noncarbonated)
   c. Unsweetened iced tea
   d. Diet soda
   e. Crystal Light
2. Eat breakfast each day. Examples of a healthy breakfast include
   a. 0.75 cup high-fiber cold cereal such as bran flakes, Fiber One, or Kashi with at least five grams of fiber or more. Serve with

0.75 cup 1 percent or skim milk and half a banana. (Participants will learn to read labels in the skills-building section to determine the amount of fiber in a cereal serving.)

  b. 1 cup cottage cheese with 1 cup fresh fruit
  c. 1 cup cooked oatmeal and one piece of fruit
  d. Two slices whole-wheat toast with one tablespoon of preserves and half a grapefruit
  e. Yogurt with fruit and granola (1 cup low-fat or fat-free yogurt, 0.5 cup of sliced fruit, two tablespoons low-fat granola, two tablespoons honey)

3. Consume 8–10 servings of fruits and vegetables each day.
  a. Have approximately 2 cups of fruit and 2.5 cups of vegetables per day.
  b. 1 serving of round fruit (apple, peach, orange) is approximately the size of a tennis ball.
  c. 1 serving of vegetables is equal to 1 cup raw vegetables or 0.5 cup cooked vegetables.

4. Consume 2–3 servings of low-fat dairy daily. This may include
  a. 1 oz. of low-fat cheese
  b. 1 cup skim milk or 1 percent milk
  c. 1 cup fat-free or low-fat yogurt

5. Limit consumption of table salt and choose lower-sodium versions of foods and condiments.

6. Consume a small portion of nuts, seeds, or legumes four to five days per week, approximately equal to 20 low-sodium nuts, two tablespoons of seeds, and 0.5 cup cooked dried beans.

7. Limit alcohol consumption to no more than one drink per day for women and two drinks per day for men.

8. Choose at least 6 servings of whole grains per day (e.g., whole-wheat bread, brown rice, whole-wheat pasta, and other whole-grain products).

9. Consume 2 servings of healthy lean protein per day such as 3-oz. portions of low-fat meats, skinless chicken, or fish.

10. Eliminate high-fat snacks.

Physical Activity/Sedentary Behavior Goals

1. Brisk walking for at least 20 minutes, six days per week, preferably in bouts of at least 10 minutes. Alternatively, participants can choose one of the following activities as a replacement:
  a. 20 minutes of bicycling about five to nine miles per hour using a stationary bike or on flat roads if bicycling outside

      b. 20 minutes of recreational swimming or water aerobics

      c. 20 minutes dancing at high intensity

      d. 20 minutes of using a stair-climber machine at a light to moderate pace

      e. 20 minutes of playing tennis

2. Reach 10,000 steps each day, increasing in increments of 2,500 steps until the 10,000 steps/day goal is reached.

3. Limit television watching to less than two hours per day.

4. Perform strength-training exercises at least two days per week.

Behavioral Goals

1. Self-monitor weight daily (at the same time each day).

2. Exercise before the day begins (e.g., work or school).

3. Avoid late-night eating after dinner (i.e., after 8:00 P.M. if you eat dinner around 6:00 P.M.).

4. Avoid fast food restaurants. If unable to avoid these restaurants, choose healthier options such as a salad with fat-free or no dressing or a fruit cup.

Medication Adherence Goals

1. Take blood pressure medication properly each day.

WHAT ABOUT HIGH-RISK GROUPS?

Be Fit, Be Well is one of few studies that focus on lower-socioeconomic-status blacks. Are there other approaches that might work? One of the hallmarks of the modern age of health research is learning from the successes of our colleagues. Body & Soul provides an excellent opportunity.

Body & Soul is a faith-based health promotion program that is focused on diet. Body & Soul is a church-based program that is designed to work with African American churches. The primary goal is to increase consumption of fruits and vegetables among church members to help reduce the risk of diet-related chronic diseases such as hypertension, heart disease, stroke, and diabetes. As we previously discussed, African Americans suffer disproportionate rates of disease and premature death from these diet- and obesity-related diseases. Most Americans, including African Americans, do not consume the recommended amounts of fruits and vegetables each day. A national survey found that only 25 percent of Americans are consuming five or more fruits and vegetables daily, and non-Hispanic blacks were less likely to meet the recommendations as compared to non-Hispanic whites (Casagrande et al. 2007). While Body & Soul is not a weight-loss intervention per se, the intervention messages are very similar to those in interventions explicitly focused on weight loss.

Why focus on African American churches for a health promotion intervention? Church, no matter what denomination, is a very important institution within African American communities. The pastor provides leadership on many levels including spiritual, social, and community-outreach issues. Attendance at church is high, especially in the southeastern United States. Members attend often and usually over a long period of time. As a result, public health workers may have more success not only in making contact with potential participants but also in tracking changes in health-related behavior over time. Finally, many churches have health committees because health is considered part of the mission of many churches (Campbell, Hudson et al. 2007).

Body & Soul is based on two successful programs that originally took place in the 1990s in churches in rural, eastern North Carolina and urban Atlanta, Georgia. Both projects resulted in an increase in fruit and vegetable consumption by about one serving a day. As a result, the most effective components of each of the two original interventions were combined for the Body & Soul effectiveness trial (Resnicow et al. 2004).

This trial had four components. First, churchwide nutrition activities were held, including a kick-off event and at least three nutrition events (e.g., taste tests, cooking demonstrations). The pastor provided support by including messages in his sermons about fruits and vegetables. Second, Body & Soul provided self-help materials, including a cookbook and nutrition video. Third, the program included a minimum of one policy or environmental change (e.g., making sure fruits and vegetables were served at church food events). Finally, the trial included peer counseling by a trained church member. This peer provided counseling and helped motivate other members to increase fruit and vegetable consumption (Campbell, Resnicow et al. 2007). The architects of Body & Soul really wanted the program to work under real-world conditions. That is, they recognized that it would not be practical to implement an intervention at multiple sites (i.e., churches) with professionally trained staff. Instead, they wanted to understand the impacts of the program as delivered by volunteer members of the churches (Resnicow et al. 2004).

A total of eight churches received the intervention while seven churches served as comparisons and completed surveys but did not receive the Body & Soul program. The churches were located in California, Georgia, North Carolina, South Carolina, Virginia, and Delaware. A total of 58 volunteer advisors in the churches administered the program and collected surveys about fruit and vegetable intake at the beginning of the program (baseline) and six months after the program had been in place. A total of 854 people completed both baseline and six-month follow-up surveys. The intervention churches had increased their fruit and vegetable consumption by 1.4 servings as compared to the comparison churches (Resnicow et al. 2004).

The Body & Soul effectiveness trial was a collaborative partnership between African American churches, the University of North Carolina, Emory University, the American Cancer Society (ACS), and the National Cancer Institute (NCI). Public health researchers at the universities provided program management while the ACS provided funding for program development and implementation (e.g., training manuals, transportation) and the NCI funded research to understand if the program worked to improve fruit and vegetable intake and the process by which it achieved its effects. And the churches benefited because they were able to pursue their health mission. All the partners were careful to consider whether all aspects of the program were culturally and spiritually suitable. For example, the cookbook included recipes submitted by church members and had to include at least one-quarter serving of fruits or vegetables per serving and be low in fat. This was an attempt to ensure that foods included in the cookbook were culturally appropriate, commonly used, and available in the community (Campbell, Hudson et al. 2007; Resnicow et al. 2004).

As a result of the improvements in fruit and vegetable consumption that occurred in the Body & Soul effectiveness trial, the NCI moved forward with its national partners the ACS and the Centers for Disease Control to disseminate the program across the United States. The program is part of an effort to decrease health disparities and increase fruit and vegetable consumption in the African American community. The program now has a group of clergy who serve as advisors to the program. Outreach to spread the word about the program is done at national meetings of clergy as well as via nonreligious groups, interfaith alliances, and radio and TV announcements that focus on African Americans. The program is designed to work without the involvement of any researchers. In addition, there is a training video that church members can watch to become peer counselors within their church. A special Web site for Body & Soul contains materials that pastors and church members can access free of charge (http://www.bodyandsoul.nih.gov). It features downloadable Body & Soul program manuals, an image library that contains pictures with a fruit and vegetable theme that may be used in church bulletins or church Web sites, and a video message from Vickie Winans, a gospel recording artist and the national Body & Soul spokesperson (Campbell, Hudson et al. 2007).

At this time, an evaluation of the national Body & Soul program is in progress. It includes a sampling of churches from across the country that have implemented the program. The results should be quite useful in determining what is required to successfully disseminate a program such as Body & Soul on a national basis.

GLOBESITY

Globesity is a term that has been used to describe the global obesity epidemic (Eberwine 2002). Obesity is not a problem that affects developed countries alone. Low-income and middle-income countries, such as China, India, Brazil, Chile, Nigeria, and Pakistan, are witnessing rapid increases in the prevalence of obesity in their populations. In fact, the rise in the prevalence of overweight and obesity in developing countries is outpacing the increase in developed countries. The number of people in the world who suffer from undernutrition has declined to 1.2 billion, while the number of people who are overnourished is approximately the same! The World Health Organization (WHO) estimates that 1 billion adults worldwide are overweight and 300 million are obese. By 2015 it is projected that 1.5 billion adults worldwide will be overweight (WHO 2005). Globalization in the form of lowered trade barriers, multinational corporations, and mass media have played a part in the globesity epidemic. Economic development and the process of modernization, industrialization, and urbanization have both positive and negative impacts on the health of populations in developing countries. In this section, we discuss the causes of the global obesity epidemic and its impact on developing countries.

The prevalence of overweight and obesity in Australia is 70.1 percent for men, 57.1 percent for women, and 29.9 percent for children; in the United Kingdom, 68.4 percent for men, 57.6 percent for women, and 25.8 percent for children; in the United States, 66.8 percent for men, 61 percent for women, and 33.2 percent for children; in Brazil, 36.2 percent for men, 38.1 percent for women, and 12.6 percent for children; in Russia, 58.4 percent for men, 47.3 percent for women, and 11.1 percent for children; in China, 26.0 percent for men, 28.5 percent for women, and 11.4 percent for children; in Vietnam, 4.4 percent for men, 6.4 percent for women, and 1.4 percent for children; and in Indonesia, 11.4 percent for men, 22.1 percent for women, and 4.0 percent for children (Popkin 2007).

Why Has the Obesity Epidemic Gone Global?

The *nutrition transition* is a phenomenon that occurs as countries globally undergo economic growth, which influences the diet of the population and leads to decreased physical activity, which in turn leads to overweight and obesity (Popkin 2005). Dr. Barry Popkin of the University of North Carolina has studied the nutrition transition and its causes for many years. When a country experiences a rapid expansion in its economy, with many workers transitioning from manual labor to more sedentary jobs in urban centers, eating styles shift. That is, people shifted from consuming traditional local foods made by traditional preparation methods to eating high-calorie processed foods that are mass produced and mass marketed. Less time is devoted to food preparation than in the past, and there is an increase in the consumption of food outside the home. Due to changes in the world food supply, there is a greater consumption of sugar, salt, fat, cholesterol, and sweetened drinks and a decrease in fiber, grain, fruit, and vegetable intake. Food that is mass marketed is cheap, and fresh foods are becoming more expensive and less accessible. Of particular note is the increase in the consumption of edible oils, energy-dense foods that are nutrient poor, and animal sources of foods (Popkin 2004, 2007a, 2007b).

Accompanying these changes in food consumption are dramatic reductions in both leisure time and occupational physical activity. As mentioned above, with economic expansion many workers depart from their work in agriculture to jobs in the service sector such as highly mechanized factories and call centers. Rather than walking or bicycling, there is an increased use of motorized transport such as motorbikes, busses, and cars. Even the energy expended at home is reduced as food preparation and household chores become increasingly mechanized due to modern devices such as food processors and washing machines (Popkin 2004).

As the socioeconomic status of a population improves, people no longer eat solely to satisfy their hunger. There is a shift to what is termed *external eating* (Hawks 2004). That is, people respond to environmental and social triggers regarding food, not just to their own hunger. For example, people may smell food in the air and decide to eat or may eat while gathered with friends even if they are not hungry. They also respond to media cues about eating. The topic of media and obesity will be discussed in the next section, but, briefly, people may be influenced to be thin by what they see on Western television or in other media. They deprive themselves of food and in response to this deprivation often eat emotionally due to anger, boredom, and frustration (Madanat et al. 2007). The result of the nutrition transition process is obesity and an increased prevalence of chronic disease.

Of particular importance is the pace at which developing countries have undergone economic transition, which results in rapid urbanization, improved socioeconomic status, and typically greater Western influence in terms of advertising and media. Countries such as China and India have become more modern and industrialized in the span of 10 to 20 years whereas the United States, Europe, and other industrialized countries experienced this transition over the span of decades to a century or more.

Jordan, a Middle Eastern country with a population of just over 6 million people, has a high prevalence of overweight along with Egypt and Mexico. Evidence that women in Jordan are depriving themselves of food and engaging in external and emotional eating suggests that this lower-middle-income country is well into its own nutrition transition (Madanat et al. 2007). Jordan has experienced significant socioeconomic growth and growth in population from 2.2 million in 1980 to 4.4 million in 1999. This growth in population is attributed to a combination of health reform, decreased infant mortality, and increased life expectancy. At the same time, the population has shifted to the cities from rural areas. However, the problem of overweight and obesity is not limited to urban areas, as it is in most countries such as Brazil, South Africa, and Turkey. In Jordan, the prevalence of overweight (body mass index [BMI] ≥ 25) among both urban and rural women between the ages of 20 to 49 years is well above 69.4 percent and 63 percent, respectively. And the prevalence of overweight is more of a problem than underweight in the rural areas of most developing countries, with the exception of Haiti, India, and some African countries including Niger, the Central African Republic, and Burkina Faso (Mendez 2005).

In Mexico between 1984 and 1998, the average purchase of fruits and vegetables in households declined by 29 percent and average soda purchases increased by 37 percent. What is happening in Mexico is a reflection of what is happening in many other developing countries: a shift in dietary intake to higher-fat food and refined carbohydrates. In Mexico, the percentage of total energy from fat increased from 23.5 percent to 30.3 percent between 1988 and 1999 (Rivera et al. 2004).

Overweight and obesity had been thought of as problems of the wealthy; however, recent data indicate this is not the case. The prevalence of obesity is higher among poorer populations. A study conducted by the Mexican National Institute of Public Health in 2000 examined overweight and obesity in relation to socioeconomic status. The prevalence of overweight and obesity increased with decreasing socioeconomic status (Rivera et al. 2004). When resources are limited, people choose less-expensive food, which is often energy dense (high in fat and refined carbohydrates) and low in nutritional value. People living in poverty may receive adequate or excessive calories, but the calories may not be from healthy food.

Chronic Disease—The Double Burden of Disease

The nutrition transition has serious health implications. The chronic diseases that arise from obesity have emerged as a major challenge to countries around the world. In recent decades, it has become apparent that developing countries that once faced problems of childhood undernutrition and infectious disease are now faced with what is known as the *double burden of disease*. While these countries continue to combat infectious diseases such as HIV/ AIDS, malaria, and tuberculosis, they are also experiencing an increase in disease and death from noninfectious or noncommunicable diseases caused by overnutrition such as type 2 diabetes, cardiovascular disease, and cancer. The WHO annual report estimated that in 2005 about 35 million out of 58 million total deaths worldwide were due to noncommunicable diseases. To put the problem of global chronic diseases into perspective, about 17 million deaths in 2005 were judged to be caused by infectious disease, about half the number thought to be caused by chronic disease. Noncommunicable diseases are also the predominant cause of death in low- and middle-income countries and were projected to account for 80 percent of all deaths and 16 million deaths in people under age 70 in these countries. Deaths by noninfectious diseases are expected to increase by 17 percent in the next 10 years. By the year 2020, it is estimated that 7 out of every 10 deaths in developing countries will be caused by noninfectious diseases versus less than 5 out of 10 today. Tobacco is a major problem and is included in these statistics.

In his introduction to the WHO (2005) report, the director-general of the WHO, Jong-wook Lee, points out that developing countries suffer more from chronic diseases because people develop these diseases at younger ages, suffer longer, and die at a lower average age as compared to people in developed countries.

The burden of obesity-related chronic diseases is likely to be more keenly felt in developing countries. These countries are less equipped to treat illness in most cases. The health systems of many poor, developing countries are already functioning on scarce resources and are not able to manage the influx of new patients and conditions. As a result, because people cannot obtain necessary preventive care or ongoing care for their illnesses, there is more disease and higher mortality rates from these diseases as compared to developed nations (Boutayeb 2006). For example, one in four people between the ages of 35 and 64 in some developing countries in the Middle East die from diabetes, whereas in developed countries diabetes affects mostly older populations (Boutayeb 2006). According to the WHO (2005), over three-quarters of diabetes-related deaths globally occur in low- and middle-income countries. This impacts the economy of these countries because the people who are of working age are falling victim to chronic diseases. In addition, the complications that arise from diabetes, in the form of blindness and infections of the extremities, increase the burden in developing countries ill-equipped to help people manage the disease (Boutayeb 2006).

Poor people in developing countries also suffer a greater burden of disease. An unfortunate and unfair truth is that poor people in developing countries do not have equal access to a healthy life. Their economic situation gives them few options regarding where they live, what food they eat, and their access to education and health care. Poor people may not fully understand the disease they are suffering from and the care it requires because they do not have access to health information. The cycle of poverty and chronic disease is predicted to be perpetuated by the obesity epidemic. In fact, the WHO report describes chronic diseases as an underappreciated cause of poverty. Obesity-related chronic disease can easily plunge a family into deeper poverty by robbing a family of its primary breadwinner and/or burdening families with the costs of medical treatment (WHO 2005).

The WHO has set up the Global Database on Body Mass Index, which is still in development (http://www.who.int/bmi/index.jsp), in order to monitor the problem of obesity around the world. They set up this database because there was not reliable national information on the prevalence of obesity in many countries. In order to develop strategies to tackle the problem of global obesity, it is important to understand the scope of the problem.

China: A Country Example of the Nutrition Transition

China has one of the largest emerging economies in the world. In the last 20 years, it has undergone rapid social and economic transformations. It is an example of a country that is in the midst of the nutrition transition. Between 1989 and 1997, the proportion of overweight or obese Chinese adults increased from 7.9 percent to 17.6 percent (Bell et al. 2001). According to the WHO (2005), 20 percent of children age 7 to 17 years in China's urban areas are overweight or obese. The current estimated prevalence of overweight and obesity among adults is 25 percent, which is still much lower than the prevalence in many Western countries. However, the percentage of adults who become obese each year is greater than in most other countries. For example, in China 1.2 percent of men became overweight or obese in each of the last 10 years versus the case in the United States, where about 0.8 percent per year became overweight or obese between 1991 and 2002 (Popkin 2008).

There has been rapid urbanization of populations in China to cities like Shanghai and smaller industrial cities. China experienced industrialization at an explosive pace as migrant workers switched from working in agriculture or other physically demanding occupations to industries in cities. Over a relatively short period of time, a large portion of the population has shifted from living and working in a more rural setting to an urban one where employment is more sedentary due to the adoption of technology in manufacturing and services. With this population shift comes lifestyle changes, including a decrease in physical activity, an increase in motorized transport, a decrease in labor-intensive work, an increase in the consumption of processed foods, more food eaten away from home, and more time using computers and watching TV. It is estimated that 95 percent of Chinese households have a TV (Popkin 2008).

Before 1980, China struggled with food shortages. Sugar was barely consumed in traditional Chinese diets; however, over time the intake of sugar and fat has increased in China. The Chinese are not alone in responding to previous eras of deprivation by indulging (James 2008). There have been major shifts in the sources of energy in the diet of the Chinese people, especially with regard to fat consumption. For example, in 1980 fat intake was 14 percent of dietary energy intake. By 1989 this figure had risen to 19.3 percent among adults age 20 to 45 years. In 1997 it was estimated that the average fat intake of young Chinese adults was 27.3 percent (Popkin 2003). In 2006 about 44 percent of the population consumed a diet that consisted of greater than 30 percent of dietary energy from fat (Popkin 2008).

Food purchases are dependent on cost, availability, and marketing. The Chinese are responding to the low cost of high-fat foods and edible oils by purchasing these products. As the production and importation of edible oils continues to increase in China, it is predicted that prices will remain low (James 2008). Energy-dense processed foods are readily available, meaning that they are accessible and affordable, in the growing number of supermarkets. And just like many other developing and developed countries, the population is influenced to purchase unhealthy foods and fast foods due to the concentrated marketing efforts of the companies that produce them (James 2008). One of the consequences of low food prices, ready availability, and intensive marketing campaigns is that there has been a shift away from traditional Chinese dietary patterns.

There has also been a rapid rise in the availability of fast food in China. Kentucky Fried Chicken (KFC) and McDonald's are the dominant chains, but they face increased competition from Chinese companies including Kungfu Catering and Malan Noodles. In 2000 there were 1,400 fast food chains in China with about 500,000 stores (*China Daily* 2008). In 1987 KFC opened its first outlet in China. Today, there are 2,500 restaurants in almost 500 cities in the Chinese mainland, and a new KFC opens in China at the rate of one per day (Yum Brands n.d.). There is even a Starbucks nestled within the walls of the Forbidden City! As we discussed earlier, the portion sizes of fast food are very large, and the meals are characterized by high calories and high fat content, including trans fat and added sugar (soft drinks).

A recent analysis from the China Health and Nutrition Survey indicated that eating patterns in China are indeed becoming less healthy. Socioeconomic status is associated with both increased consumption of snack food and overconsumption of fried food. Cooking practices are also changing from boiling or steaming food to frying it. Urban populations were found to engage in more snacking and overconsumption of fried food as compared to residents of rural areas (Z. Wang et al. 2008).

The daily demands on energy expenditure associated with the changes in lifestyle in China due to economic expansion have decreased by an estimated 400 to 800 kcal/day. People have not reduced their food consumption in response to decreased physical activity. Living in an urban environment and the changes in working and living conditions were estimated to decrease daily energy expenditure by 300 to 400 kcal/day. Using a bicycle for transportation to work (assuming it takes an hour each way) would amount to an energy expenditure of 480 kcal/day. Since people are transitioning to motorized forms of transport, riding public transit would require an energy expenditure of 316 kcal/day and driving would expend only 200 kcal/day. To make up for the difference in energy expenditure between driving and biking (280 kcal), a person would have to walk for 80 minutes. It is estimated that the average Chinese person is gaining 0.5 kg per year in added weight as there is no longer enough physical activity in his or her daily routine to offset this gain (James 2008).

What Can Be Done to Tackle the Problem of Global Obesity?

It is not likely that the globesity epidemic can be stopped. However, there are some steps that have been suggested that may be able to slow the pace of the epidemic. One suggestion has been to introduce food labeling, which would involve requiring a red, yellow, or green label on foods that contain high, moderate, or low levels of fat, sugar, and salt. Trade restrictions in the form of taxes on imported unhealthy foods have been proposed. Taxes on unhealthy foods and subsidies for healthy foods such as fruits and vegetables to make them more affordable have also been suggested. Increasing the availability of healthy food choices by working with local farms to bring produce into the cities has been advocated, as has the prohibition of food marketing to children. Denmark took a proactive step in 2003 by introducing a law restricting the amount of trans-fatty acids in food products to a maximum of 2 percent of fat content. The law provided for punishment in the form of prison time if the law was violated (Astrup 2008).

On the surface, the explanation for high rates of obesity is the same in developed and developing countries. Put simply, there have been changes in dietary patterns and levels of physical activity. However, every country in the world has its own culture, traditions, history, and politics, which also play into how the epidemic rears its head in each country. The improved economic conditions in many developing countries mean that the population becomes more affluent, food is more readily available, there is a shift to less labor-intensive work, and people have a more sedentary lifestyle. Countries undergoing this shift experience a nutrition transition that results in obesity and rising levels of chronic disease in the population. Durable solutions must be put in place to prevent the epidemic from growing any more than it has already.

MEDIA AND OBESITY

What is media? The definition of media continues to expand. Types of media include television, movies, radio, video games, cell phones, print media (e.g., newspapers, magazines), music, the Internet, and advertising. The list will doubtless continue to expand as more new technology moves into the marketplace and is adopted by greater numbers of people. As a result of the increasing interest in media, research on how people use media in different ways is sure to expand. For example, many people now read the newspaper online or on handheld devices such as smart phones (e.g., iPhone, Black-Berry). In addition to providing us with news, entertainment, and information, media also influence how we think and the purchases we make.

The American Academy of Pediatrics recommends that children have two or fewer hours of screen time per day, which includes television, DVD watching, playing video games, or computer time. The reality is that the average amount of time children spend using media is five and a half hours per day (Kaiser Family Foundation 2004). It is estimated that children between the ages of 2 and 11 watch an average of three hours of television a day (Gantz et al. 2007). In fact, almost 36 percent of preschoolers have more than two hours of screen time (TV/video and computer use) per day (Mendoza 2007).

It is believed that excess exposure to media in youth has immediate negative health effects and will lead to negative health consequences in adulthood. Researchers in New Zealand followed 1,000 kids until they reached age 26 in order to examine the relationship between childhood TV viewing and adult health. TV viewing in childhood and adolescence predicted higher BMIs in adulthood (Hancox 2004). Despite this compelling evidence, this is a relatively new area of research, and we do not yet have enough data to draw firm conclusions. Most studies of the topic have been conducted in children and consider children's programming. However, many children also watch programming meant for adults. Most research studies in this area have focused on the relationship between obesity and one form of media, television. It may be that other types of media such as cell phones and video games are used in different ways and therefore have different impacts. So it is hard to extrapolate from the studies done so far to suggest the mechanism by which media at large affect children's body fatness (Boyce 2007). There are several hypotheses about why media may result in childhood overweight. Screen time may promote sedentary behavior, or it may be that food advertising influences what children eat and increases total energy intake. We will explore the evidence for each of these hypotheses.

Sedentary Behavior

Time spent watching TV or playing computer games has been hypothesized to displace the time that children could spend playing outside or engaging in other physical activity. This hypothesis has not been proven by studies on the topic. For example, a meta-analysis, a study in which all the data on a particular area of research are gathered together and reanalyzed, demonstrated that the small relationship between TV viewing, video/computer game use, and body fatness could be explained by factors other than TV viewing and video/computer game use (Marshall 2004). The same study also found only a small relationship between TV viewing, video/computer game use, and moderate and vigorous physical activity. In other words, factors other than TV viewing alone, such as consumption of unhealthy snacks while watching TV, should be considered in the TV viewing–body fatness relationship (Marshall 2004).

The relationship between TV viewing, interactive media (Internet surfing and video games), and body fat and BMI was examined in female high school students. The girls answered questions about their physical activity patterns and rode a special bicycle that measured cardiovascular fitness. The height and weight of the girls was measured to determine BMI, and percentage of body fat was measured via dual-energy x-ray absorptiometry. This study was unique in that it examined two types of media, interactive and noninteractive (e.g., TV, videos, and movies). TV was not found to be correlated with body fat or BMI. However, interactive media were found to be correlated with body fat and BMI independent of participation in moderate or vigorous physical activity and cardiovascular fitness. In other words, the hypothesis that the time spent using interactive media is related to body fat or BMI by displacing physical activity was not found to be true in this study (Schneider 2007).

A national study of preschool children (ages 2 to 5 years) found that watching more than two hours of TV or videos per day was independently related to increased risk of overweight (BMI-for-age $\geq$ 85th and < 95th percentiles), obesity (BMI-for-age > 95th percentile), and higher adiposity (measured by skinfold thickness) as compared to watching TV two hours or less per day. The study also found that any computer use (more than zero hours per day) among preschoolers was related to higher adiposity as compared to no computer use (Mendoza 2007). The positive findings regarding the association between TV/video and computer use in relation to adiposity from this study among preschoolers indicate that children's age may affect the relationship between media and obesity.

Food Advertisements and Marketing to Children

Food advertisements are aired during children's TV programming and heavily promote candy, fast foods, and sugary cereals, thus influencing children's eating behavior and food choice. In fact, food is the most commonly advertised product in children's television programming (Boyce 2007). The most commonly advertised foods types are candy and snacks (34 percent of food advertisements), cereal (28 percent), and fast food restaurants (10 percent). In contrast, only 4 percent of food ads were for dairy products, 1 percent for fruit juice, and none for fruits and vegetables (Gantz et al. 2007). Children, especially those under the age of 8, may not recognize that advertisers employ persuasive tactics to get them to choose certain foods (Kunkel et al. 2004). In other words, kids are unable to critically think about the messages that are being delivered via these advertisements, so they may take advertising claims at face value.

What types of foods are being advertised to children? What is the nutritional value of these foods? And what are the strategies and messages utilized in the marketing of these foods to children? One study sought to answer these questions by analyzing advertisements for food that were aired during Saturday morning children's TV programs. Researchers recorded 27.5 hours of Saturday morning children's TV programming from many different channels broadcast in Washington, D.C., over the course of one month. Of all the advertisements, almost half (49 percent) were for food. The proportion of food advertisements that were for foods high in fat, with added sugars or sodium, was 91 percent! Only 7 percent of advertisements were for foods that contained at least half a serving of fruits and vegetables. The most popular marketing techniques utilized in Saturday morning children's TV programming were some type of character (e.g., movie character, character in costume) (74 percent), giveaways (26 percent), encouragement to visit the product Web site or use its e-mail address (15 percent), and animation (15 percent). Some advertisements employed a few of the techniques together in the same advertisement. The food advertisements were misleading because they would often include messages about health or physical activity, but the foods advertised were inherently unhealthy. For example, we often see advertisements for cereals high in sugar and hear the narrator of the commercial say, "part of a nutritious breakfast." Last, 86 percent of the food advertisements appealed to children's emotions by including messages relating the product to being fun or cool (Batada et al. 2008).

The budget for public service announcements (PSAs) about the merits of healthy foods such as fruits, vegetables, and whole grains is very meager in comparison to the ad budgets of food companies. Food manufacturers spent $7 billion in 1997 on advertising, and 75 percent of the budget for advertising for food manufacturers was spent on television advertising. The proportion of the advertising budget spent on TV advertising was even higher for the fast food industry: 95 percent (Gallo 1999).

One study examined over 1,600 hours of children's television programming and confirmed that children see thousands of food advertisements each year. For example, children age 2–7 years saw over 12 food ads per day, which amounts to over 4,400 ads per year; "tweens" age 8–12 years saw 21 food ads per day and over 7,600 per year; teenagers age 13–17 years saw 17 food ads per day and over 6,000 per year. PSAs promoting physical activity or nutrition were rarely seen in comparison to food advertisements. For example, children under 8 years old saw one PSA for every 26 food advertisements, tweens saw one PSA for every 48 food ads, and teenagers saw one PSA for every 130 food ads (Gantz et al. 2007).

Some large food companies including Kraft, General Mills, and Kellogg have adopted nutrition standards similar to the recommendations of health experts in deciding what foods they will market to children. And some companies, including those mentioned above, have made the choice not to direct advertisements to children under the age of 6 (Batada et al. 2008). Great Britain has banned the advertisement of foods high in sugar, salt, and fat to children age 16 and under and the use of cartoon characters, contests, or sweepstakes in ads during children's TV shows (Gantz et al. 2007).

Increased Consumption

Another hypothesis is that children do not pay attention to what they eat or how much they eat because they are distracted by media. One study found that increasing screen time by 50 percent was related to an increase in energy intake of 250 kcal/day among a group of nonobese 8- to 12-year-olds (Epstein et al. 2002).

Increased time spent watching television is related to decreased intake of fruits and vegetables in adolescents (Boynton-Jarrett et al. 2003). This information, along with the knowledge that television viewing increases the consumption of unhealthy foods commonly advertised on TV, seems to suggest that the influence of food advertisements is a factor in these relationships.

A study followed 548 sixth and seventh graders for almost 20 months to track how much time students spent watching television, total caloric intake, and consumption of foods frequently advertised on TV. At the beginning of the study, researchers measured the height and weight of the students. Each student filled out a survey that asked questions about his or her levels of physical activity, food intake, and time spent watching television. The researchers were particularly interested in the intake of foods commonly advertised on television (FCAT), which included sugar-sweetened beverages (e.g., soda, Kool-Aid), salty snacks (e.g., potato chips), fried potatoes, sweet baked snacks (e.g., cookies, Pop-Tarts), candy, and fast food meals. Increased television viewing was associated with an increase in total calorie intake. For every additional hour of television the students watched, their total energy intake increased by 167 kcal/day. In addition, the researchers found that increases of television viewing were associated with increased consumption of FCAT by 0.2 to 1.4 servings per week. In summary, these students consumed more calories when they were watching TV, and they consumed more calories from unhealthy foods commonly advertised on TV (Wiecha et al. 2006).

Does Decreasing Children's Screen Time Lead to Weight Loss?

The answer to the question posed above is generally yes. However, these studies also investigated other behaviors, so it is difficult to examine the role of decreased screen time on weight loss in isolation. The following study did look solely at reducing screen time. Researchers assigned children ages two to seven years old who had BMIs ≥ 75th percentile for age and sex to two different groups and tracked them for two years. The first group (intervention group) had their TV viewing and computer use reduced by 50 percent; the second group (control group) had no change in their TV viewing and computer use. The children in the intervention group decreased their sedentary behavior, decreased their energy intake, and decreased their BMIs as compared to the control group. The study also demonstrated that the results may be due more to the decrease in energy intake rather than any changes in physical activity (Epstein et al. 2008).

The Center for Media and Child Health at Children's Hospital Boston is involved in researching the effects of media on child health. The center compiles a database of any research published in the area of media and child health; summarizes it in plain language; and makes it available to parents, teachers, and researchers (http://cmch.tv). In addition, the center's Web site provides helpful information and tips on how to use or experience the different forms of media in healthy ways for children of all ages such as setting limits on screen time, coviewing (parents and children watching TV or movies together), and teaching media literacy. In other words, it provides information to teachers, parents, and researchers on how to be savvy media consumers.

WHAT DOES THE FUTURE HOLD?

The obesity research field is filled with examples of impressive successes but also many disappointments. As the amount of money available for research has dwindled and competition for those funds has increased, researchers have worked hard to maximize the efforts and money expended. As a result, the interventions to prevent and treat obesity have become more refined. Unfortunately, the research dollars spent have been no match for the larger forces in society, from changes in the physical environment to the huge amounts of money spent marketing junk food. As a result, rates of overweight and obesity remain high.

Timeline

23,000–25,000 BCE	Paleolithic artifacts of obese figures are created in Europe and the Middle East.
5th century BCE	Hippocrates suggests "hard work" before food for treating obesity.
2nd century CE	Galen identifies moderate and immoderate obesity.
16th century	Nicholas Bonetus dissects an obese person.
1614	Santorio describes his metabolic scale for measuring changes in the body as a function of metabolic processes.
1752	Réaumur writes on the digestion of food.
18th century	Lazzaro Spallanzani demonstrates that gastric liquid digests food.
1830s	Sylvester Graham gains a following and advocates eating brown bread.

1833–1838	William Beaumont publishes his description of the digestive process based on his observations of Alexis St. Martin.
1835	Quetelet describes his index for body mass.
1863	William Banting publishes the first popular diet book.
1879	Hoggan and Hoggan outline the growth and development of fat cells.
1880	Dr. Tanner begins his famous fast.
1880s	J. H. Kellogg takes over running the Battle Creek Sanitarium.
1889	The first modern lipectomy is performed.
1893	Thyroid extract is used to treat obesity.
1896	The first human calorimeter is constructed at Wesleyan University in Connecticut.
1898	Horace Fletcher loses over 40 pounds and begins a mastication movement.
19th century	Justus von Liebig identifies carbohydrate, protein, and fat.
1901	The New York Life Insurance Company reports that overweight men have higher mortality rates.
1902	Russell Chittenden begins studies on the number of calories needed by humans and the minimal amount of protein on which a person can function.
1904	Lane Bryant opens her first store.
1922	A gene causing obesity in mice is identified.
1923	Charles Davenport notes the heritability of obesity in families.
1963	An association between socioeconomic status and obesity is documented.
1970	Mason and Ito perform their gastric bypass surgery.
1972	*Dr. Atkins' Diet Revolution* is published.
1994	The leptin gene is cloned.
1997	Fen-phen is taken off the market after significant side effects are documented, including several deaths.

2004   The American Cancer Society publishes a landmark study of over 900,000 people linking excess body weight to increased risk of death from cancer.

2006   The New York City Board of Health votes to ban trans fats in restaurants.

2008   Two-thirds of U.S. adults are overweight or obese; one-third of U.S. adults are obese.

Glossary

Abdominal fat Adipose tissue that is centrally distributed between the thorax and pelvis.

Adipose tissue Fat cells in the body.

Atherosclerosis Deposits of fatty substances and calcium in the lining of arteries that result in narrowing of the arteries. Hardening of the arteries may occur in older individuals.

Bariatric surgery An umbrella term for several gastric operations that help promote weight loss among severely obese individuals.

Basal metabolic rate (BMR) Energy spent by an individual while at rest.

Biliopancreatic diversion A type of bariatric surgery that combines a reduction in the size of the stomach with the construction of bypasses of segments of the small intestines.

Body composition Usually measured as the percentage of fat mass and fat-free mass (muscle, bone, water, tissues) in the body.

Body image Personal conception of one's own body as distinct from one's actual anatomic body or the conception other people have of it.

Body mass index (BMI) Body weight in kilograms divided by the height in meters squared (wt/ht^2).

Bulimia (bulimia nervosa) A type of eating disorder involving binge eating followed by self-induced vomiting, use of laxatives or diuretics, fasting, or vigorous exercise in order to prevent weight gain; often accompanied by feelings of guilt, depression, or self-disgust.

Calorie A unit of energy.

Calorimeter An apparatus for measuring the amount of heat released in a chemical reaction.

Cancer Diseases in which abnormal cells divide without control and are able to invade other tissues.

Carbohydrates A class of compounds containing carbon, hydrogen, and oxygen mostly created by plants. Also a class of food.

Cardiovascular disease (CVD) Any abnormal condition characterized by dysfunction of the heart, blood vessels, or circulation. CVD includes atherosclerosis, cerebrovascular disease (e.g., stroke), and hypertension.

Central adiposity See *abdominal fat*.

Central fat distribution Body fat that is concentrated around the waist and upper abdominal area.

Cholesterol A type of fat that circulates in the blood. Made by the body and found in foods of animal origin.

Chronic disease A disease that lasts for three months or longer.

Comorbidity Two or more diseases or conditions existing together in an individual.

Coronary heart disease (CHD) A type of heart disease caused by narrowing (due to the buildup of fatty deposits) of the coronary arteries that feed the heart.

Diabetes (diabetes mellitus) A group of disorders that influence how the body utilizes blood sugar (blood glucose).

Direct costs of obesity The cost of preventing, diagnosing, or treating obesity or obesity-related conditions like coronary heart disease.

Dual-energy x-ray absorptiometry (DXA) A method used to estimate total body fat and percentage of body fat.

Dyslipidemia Disorders in the lipoprotein metabolism; classified as hypercholesterolemia, hypertriglyceridemia, combined hyperlipidemia, and low levels of high-density lipoprotein (HDL) cholesterol.

Emotional eating Consuming food in response to feelings instead of hunger.

Energy dense Foods that provide a lot of calories for a given volume of food, such as candy and sugar-sweetened beverages.

Ephedrine Drug that is found in some herbal weight-loss supplements that decreases feelings of hunger. Has been found to have dangerous side effects including irregular heartbeats, high blood pressure, stroke, and death in some cases.

Ethnic disparities Variations between racial and ethnic groups in terms of a particular factor such as the prevalence of obesity or number of people suffering from a particular disease.

Fad diets A temporarily popular diet designed to cause weight loss often by eliminating entire food groups. While on the diet people may experience weight loss, but once the diet is stopped dramatic weight gain occurs. Claims of these diets are often too good to be true.

Fat A greasy, soft-solid material found in animal tissues and many plants. Serves as a form of energy storage and is an essential component of the human diet.

Gastric banding Surgery to limit the amount of food that can be comfortably consumed by placing a band around the esophagus where it meets the stomach.

Gastric bypass A surgical procedure that combines a reduction in the size of the stomach with the creation of pouches to restrict food intake and the construction of bypasses of segments of the small intestine.

Gastroesophageal reflux Regurgitation of the contents of the stomach into the esophagus.

Genetic mutation A permanent change in the DNA sequence that makes up a gene, which is the basic physical and functional unit of heredity.

Glycemic index (GI) A ranking of the rise in serum glucose from various foodstuffs.

Gout A form of arthritis that occurs suddenly and causes pain and swelling in the joints (usually the big toe) and is caused by abnormally high levels of uric acid in the bloodstream.

High-density lipoproteins (HDL) A type of "good" cholesterol. Lipoproteins that contain a small amount of cholesterol and carry cholesterol away from body cells and tissues to the liver for excretion from the body.

Hormone A chemical substance formed in one organ or part of the body and carried in the blood to another organ or part that often has a stimulating effect.

Hyperglycemia Elevated levels of glucose in the bloodstream.

Hyperinsulinemia Elevated levels of insulin in the bloodstream.

Hypertension High blood pressure.

Incidence The rate at which a certain event occurs (i.e., the number of new cases of a specific disease that occur during a certain period of time).

Indirect costs of obesity The decrease in economic activity that is associated with diseases or early death that can be blamed on obesity.

Infectious disease A disease caused by microorganisms (bacteria, viruses, fungi) that enter the body then grow and multiply there.

Insulin A hormone secreted by the pancreas that allows the body to convert blood glucose into energy.

Insulin resistance Impairment of the normal response of muscle and other cells to insulin.

Ketosis Occurs when the body begins to break down fat for energy due to not enough insulin in the body. Results in the production of toxic acids (ketones) and may cause unconsciousness or death.

Lipoprotein Molecules consisting of protein and fat that carry cholesterol, triglycerides, and other fats through the bloodstream. There are four general classes: high density, low density, very low density, and chylomicrons.

Low-density lipoprotein (LDL) A type of "bad" cholesterol. LDL carries cholesterol to the tissues of the body, including the arteries.

Macronutrients Nutrients required by the human body in the greatest amount, such as carbohydrates, protein, and fats.

Macrophage A type of white blood cell involved in the immune response of the body that ingests (takes in) foreign material.

Media literacy The ability to think critically about media messages that are designed to inform, entertain, and advertise.

Metabolic syndrome A group of conditions (high blood pressure, elevated insulin levels, unhealthy cholesterol levels, abdominal fat) that occur together to increase the risk of heart disease, stroke, and diabetes.

Morbid Affected with or induced by disease.

Nutrition transition A phenomenon that occurs as a country undergoes economic growth, which in turn influences the diet of the population and leads to decreased physical activity, which leads to overweight and obesity.

Obesity The condition of having an abnormally high proportion of body fat. Defined as a body mass index (BMI) of greater than or equal to 30.

Obesogenic Conditions or factors that lead people to become obese.

Osteoarthritis Arthritis characterized by erosion of joint cartilage. Affects mainly weight-bearing joints.

Pancreas A gland in the abdomen that secretes pancreatic juice that is discharged into the intestine and the internal secretions insulin and glucagon.

Pharmacotherapy The use of appetite-suppressant medications to manage obesity by decreasing appetite or increasing the feeling of satiety.

Placebo An inert substance given as a medicine for its suggestive effect.

Prediabetes Blood glucose levels that are higher than normal but not yet high enough to be diagnosed as diabetes.

Prevalence The number of events, such as instances of a given disease or other condition, in a specific population at a designated time.

Protein A class of compounds composed of linked amino acids that contain carbon, hydrogen, nitrogen, oxygen, and sometimes other atoms in specific configurations.

Refined carbohydrates Foods such as pasta and white bread that have gone through machinery that strips the bran and the germ from the whole grain. Such food is finer in texture and has a longer shelf life, but the process also removes important nutrients.

Roux-en-Y bypass The most common gastric bypass procedure, in which a small pouch is created at the top of the stomach and a bypass is constructed from the stomach to the lower intestine so that fewer calories are absorbed during digestion.

Satiety The quality or state of being fed to fullness.

Screen time Time spent utilizing electronic media such as television, computers, and videos (DVDs).

Sleep apnea A serious, potentially life-threatening breathing disorder in which breathing stops and starts repeatedly during sleep due to either the collapse of the upper airway or failure of the brain to send signals telling the body to breath.

Stroke An interruption of the blood supply to the brain that may be caused by a clot in (thrombosis) or rupture of (hemorrhage) a blood vessel to the brain.

Subcutaneous fat Fat under the skin.

Thyroid gland An endocrine gland located in the neck that secretes thyroid hormone and calcitonin.

Triglyceride A type of fat in the bloodstream and fat tissue. It comes from the food we eat and is also made by the body.

Type 1 diabetes (insulin-dependent diabetes mellitus) A disease characterized by the inability of the pancreas to produce adequate amounts of insulin, which results in high blood glucose. Seen mostly in younger people. Typically treated with insulin injections.

Type 2 diabetes (non–insulin-dependent diabetes mellitus) A disease in which the body becomes resistant to the effects of insulin or the pancreas does not produce enough insulin, which results in hyperglycemia and hyperinsulinemia. Typically treated with oral medications, diet, and physical activity.

Vertical banded gastroplasty A surgical treatment for extreme obesity; an operation on the stomach that involves constructing a small pouch in the stomach that empties through a narrow opening into the lower stomach and small intestine.

Very low-density lipoprotein (VLDL) Molecules that initially leave the liver, carrying cholesterol and lipid.

Visceral fat Fat located in and around the organs; belly fat.

Vitality Physical or mental vigor.

Vitamins A group of organic substances present in very small amounts in natural food and essential to normal metabolism.

Waist circumference The distance around the natural waist.

Waist-to-hip ratio (WHR) The ratio of the distance around the waist to the distance around the hips.

Bibliography

Adler J. 2008, July 7–14. "The obese should have to pay more for airline tickets." *Newsweek*. Available at: http://www.newsweek.com/id/143790.

Allison DB, Fontaine KR, Manson JE, Stevens J, VanItallie TB. 1999. "Annual deaths attributable to obesity in the United States." *JAMA* 282: 1530–1538.

Alvy LM, Calvert SL. 2008. "Food marketing on popular children's Web sites: a content analysis." *J Am Diet Assoc* 108: 710–713.

American Academy of Pediatrics. 1999. "Media Education." *Pediatrics* 104: 341–342. Available at: http://aappolicy.aappublications.org/cgi/content/full/pediatrics%3B104/2/341.

American Dietetic Association. 2006. "Position of the American Dietetic Association: individual-, family-, school-, and community-based interventions for pediatric overweight." *J Am Diet Assoc* 106: 925–945.

Andreyeva T, Sturm R, Ringel JS. 2004. "Moderate and severe obesity have large differences in health care costs." *Obes Res* 12: 1936–1943.

Arias MA, Alonso-Fernandez A, Garcia-Rio F, Pagola C. 2005. "Association between obesity and obstructive sleep apnea." *Eur Heart J* 26: 2744–2745.

Aronne, L. 2002. "Treatment of obesity in the primary care setting." In: Wadden TA, Stunkard AJ, eds. *Handbook of obesity treatment*. New York: Guilford, 383–394.

Astrup A. 2008. "Nutrition transition and its relationship to the development of obesity and related chronic diseases." *Obes Rev* 9(Suppl 1): 48–52.

Astrup A, Larsen TM, Harper A. 2004. "Atkins and other low-carbohydrate diets: hoax or an effective tool for weight loss?" *Lancet* 364: 897–899.

Banting W. 1863. *Letter on corpulence, addressed to the public.* London: Harrison. Available at: http://books.google.com/books?hl=en&id=1gA4rau7kd8C&dq=banting+Letter+on+Corpulence&printsec=frontcover&source=web&ots=JCSqMVFsIY&sig=drfZGr_2rAMgHIAAHLE-ZQ6RjoE&sa=X&oi=book_result&resnum=10&ct=result#PPP1,M1.

Barlow SE. 2007. "Expert committee recommendations regarding the prevention, assessment, and treatment of child and adolescent overweight and obesity: summary report." *Pediatrics* 120(Suppl 4): S164–192.

Barrett D. 2007. *Waistland.* New York: W.W. Norton.

Batada A, Seitz MD, Wootan MG, Story M. 2008. "Nine out of 10 food advertisements shown during Saturday morning children's television programming are for foods high in fat, sodium, or added sugars, or low in nutrients." *J Am Diet Assoc* 108: 673–678.

Beaumont W. 1838. *Experiments and observations on the gastric juice and the physiology of digestion.* Edinburgh, UK: Maclachlan & Stewart.

Bell C, Ge K, Popkin BM. 2001. "Weight gain and its predictors in Chinese adults." *Int J Obes* 25: 1079–1086.

Bertakis KD, Azari R. 2005. "Obesity and the use of health care services." *Obes Res* 13: 372–379.

Bialik C. 2008, August 15. "Obesity study looks thin." *Wall Street Journal.* Available at: http://online.wsj.com/article/SB121876145236142929.html?mod=fpa_editors_picks. Accessed January 23, 2009.

Blanck HM, Khan LK, Serdula MK. 2004. "Prescription weight loss pill use among Americans: patterns of pill use and lessons learned from the fen-phen market withdrawal." *Prev Med* 39: 1243–1248.

Body & Soul Web site. Available at: http://www.bodyandsoul.nih.gov. Accessed November 2008.

Boutayeb A. 2006. "The double burden of communicable and non-communicable diseases in developing countries." *Trans R Soc Trop Med Hyg* 100: 191–199.

Boyce T. 2007. "The media and obesity." *Obes Rev* 8(Suppl 1): 201–205.

Boynton-Jarrett R, Thomas TN, Peterson KE, Wiecha J, Sobol AM, Gortmaker SL. 2003. "Impact of television viewing patterns on fruit and vegetable consumption among adolescents." *Pediatrics* 112: 1321–1326.

Bray GA. 2002. "Drug treatment of obesity." In: Wadden TA, Stunkard AJ, eds. *Handbook of obesity treatment.* New York: Guilford, 317–338.

Bray GA. 2004. "Historical framework for the development of ideas about obesity." In: Bray GA, Bouchard C, eds. *Handbook of obesity: etiology and pathophysiology.* 2nd ed. New York: Marcel Dekker, 1–32.

Bray GA, Bouchard C. 2004. *Handbook of obesity: etiology and pathophysiology.* 2nd ed. New York: Marcel Dekker.

Bray GA, Bouchard C. 2008. *Handbook of obesity: clinical applications.* 3rd ed. New York: Informa Healthcare.

Burns CM, Tijhuis MA, Seidell JC. 2001. "The relationship between quality of life and perceived body weight and dieting history in Dutch men and women." *Int J Obes* 25: 1386–1392.

Calle EE, Rodriguez C, Walker-Thurmond K, Thun MJ. 2003. "Overweight, obesity, and mortality from cancer in a prospectively studied cohort of U.S. adults." *N Engl J Med* 348: 1625–1638.

Calle EE, Thun MJ, Petrelli JM, Rodriguez C, Heath CW Jr. 1999. "Body-mass index and mortality in a prospective cohort of U.S. adults." *N Engl J Med* 341: 1097–1105.

Campbell MK, Hudson MA, Resnicow K, Blakeney N, Paxton A, Baskin M. 2007. "Church-based health promotion interventions: evidence and lessons learned." *Annu Rev Public Health* 28: 213–234.

Campbell MK, Resnicow K, Carr C, Wang T, Williams A. 2007. "Process evaluation of an effective church-based diet intervention: Body & Soul." *Health Educ Behav* 34: 864–880.

Casagrande SS, Wang Y, Anderson C, Gary TL. 2007. "Have Americans increased their fruit and vegetable intake? The trends between 1988 and 2002." *Am J Prev Med* 32: 257–263.

Cawley J. 2004. "The impact of obesity on wages." J Human Res 39: 451–474.

Centers for Disease Control and Prevention. 2005. "Competitive foods and beverages available for purchase in secondary schools—selected sites, United States 2004." *MMWR Morb Mortal Wkly Rep* 54: 917–921.

Centers for Disease Control and Prevention. 2008a. *National diabetes fact sheet: general information and national estimates on diabetes in the United States, 2007.* Atlanta, GA: U.S. Department of Health and Human Services/Author.

Centers for Disease Control and Prevention. 2008b. "State-specific incidence of diabetes among adults—participating states, 1995–1997 and 2005–2007." *MMWR Morb Mortal Wkly Rep* 57: 1169–1173. Available at: http://www.cdc.gov/mmwr/preview/mmwrhtml/mm5743a2.htm. Accessed November 19, 2008.

Chan JM, Rimm EB, Colditz GA, Stampfer MJ, Willett WC. 1994. "Obesity, fat distribution, and weight gain as risk factors for clinical diabetes in men." *Diabetes Care* 17: 961–969.

China Daily. 2008, June 30. "Competition gearing up in China's fast food industry." Available at: http://www.chinadaily.com.cn/bizchina/2008-06/30/content_6806904_3.htm. Accessed December 2008.

Christian M. 2003, December 15. "Surgeon Dr. Mal Fobi revolutionizes weight-loss surgery with 'Fobi-Pouch Operation for Obesity.'" *Jet.* Available at: http://findarticles.com/p/articles/mi_m1355/is_25_104/ai_111616875/print.   Accessed June 2, 2008.

Cohen DA. 2008. "Reengineering the built environment: schools, worksites, neighborhoods and parks." In: Bray GA, Bouchard C, eds. *Handbook of obesity: clinical applications.* 3rd ed. New York: Informa Healthcare, 195–208.

Colditz G. 1993. "Economic costs of obesity and inactivity." *Med Sci Sports Exerc* 31: S663–S667.

Colditz GA, Willett WC, Rotnitzky A, Manson JE. 1995. "Weight gain as a risk factor for clinical diabetes mellitus in women." *Ann Intern Med* 122: 481–486.

Colman E. 2005. "Anorectics on trial: a half century of federal regulation of prescription appetite suppressants." *Ann Intern Med* 143: 380–385.

Crawford D, Jeffery RW. 2005. *Obesity prevention and public health.* New York: Oxford University Press.

Critser G. 2003. *Fat land: how Americans became the fattest people in the world.* Boston: Houghton Mifflin.

Daviglus ML, Liu K, Yan LL, Pirzada A, Manheim L, Manning W, et al. 2004. "Relation of body mass index in young adulthood and middle age to Medicare expenditures in old age." *JAMA* 292: 2743–2749.

Davis A. 2007. "An association between asthma and BMI in adolescents: results from the California Health Kids Survey." *J Asthma* 44: 873–879.

Day JC. 2008. "Population profile of the United States: national population projections." Available at: http://www.census.gov/population/www/pop-profile/natproj.html.

Delany J. 1909. "Gluttony." *Catholic encyclopedia.* Available at: http://www.newadvent.org/cathen/06590a.htm.

DiPietro L, Kohl HW III, Barlow CE, Blair SN. 1998. "Improvements in cardiorespiratory fitness attenuate age-related weight gain in healthy men and women: the Aerobics Center Longitudinal Study." *Int J Obes Relat Metab Disord* 22: 55–62.

Doggrell SA. 2006. "Sibutramine for obesity in adolescents." *Expert Opin Pharmacother* 7: 2435–2438.

Drewnowski A, Darmon N. 2005. "Food choices and diet costs: an economic analysis." *J Nutr* 135: 900–904.

Dunican KC, Desilets AR, Montalbano JK. 2007. "Pharmacotherapeutic options for overweight adolescents." *Ann Pharmacother* 41: 1445–1455.

Ebbeling CB, Leidig MM, Feldman HA, Lovesky MM, Ludwig DS. 2007. "Effects of a low-glycemic load vs low-fat diet in obese young adults." *JAMA* 297: 2092–2102.

Eberwine D. 2002. "Globesity: the crisis of growing proportions." *Perspect Health* 7(3). Available at: http://www.paho.org/English/DPI/Number15_article2_5.htm. Accessed November 2008.

Eliassen AH, Colditz GA, Rosner B, Willett WC, Hankinson SE. 2006. "Adult weight change and risk of postmenopausal breast cancer." *JAMA* 296: 193–201.

Epstein LH, Paluch RA, Consalvi A, Riordan K, Scholl T. 2002. "Effects of manipulating sedentary behavior on physical activity and food intake." *J Pediatr* 140: 334–339.

Epstein LH, Roemmich JN, Robinson JL, Paluch RA, Winiewicz DD, Fuerch JH, et al. 2008. "A randomized trial of the effects of reducing television viewing and computer use on body mass index in young children." *Arch Pediatr Adolesc Med* 162: 239–245.

Fairburn CG, Brownell KD, eds. 2005. *Eating disorders and obesity: a comprehensive handbook.* 2nd ed. New York: Guilford.

Fine JT, Colditz GA, Coakley EH, Mosely G, Manson JE, Willett WC, Kawachi I. 1999. "A prospective study of weight change and health-related quality of life in women." *JAMA* 282: 2136–42.

Finkelstein EA, Fiebelkorn IC, Wang G. 2004. "State-level estimates of annual medical expenditures attributable to obesity." *Obes Res* 12: 18–24.

Finkelstein EA, Trogdon JG, Brown DS, Allaire BT, Dellea PS, Kamal-Bahl SJ. 2008. "The lifetime medical cost burden of overweight and obesity: implications for obesity prevention." *Obesity* 16: 1843–1848.

Flegal KM, Graubard BI, Williamson DF, Gail MH. 2005. "Excess deaths associated with underweight, overweight, and obesity." *JAMA* 293: 1861–1867.

Flegal KM, Graubard BI, Williamson DF, Gail MH. 2007. "Cause-specific excess deaths associated with underweight, overweight, and obesity." *JAMA* 298: 2028–2037.

Flegal KM, Williamson DF, Pamuk ER, Rosenberg HM. 2004. "Estimating deaths attributable to obesity in the United States." *Am J Public Health* 94: 1486–1489.

Fobi MA, Lee H, Holness R, Cabinda D. 1998. "Gastric bypass operation for obesity." *World J Surg* 22: 925–935.

Ford ES. 2005. "The epidemiology of obesity and asthma." *J Allergy Clin Immunol* 115: 897–909.

Foster GD, Sherman S, Borradaile KE, Grundy KM, Vander Veur SS, Nachmani J, et al. 2008. "A policy-based school intervention to prevent overweight and obesity." *Pediatrics* 121: e794–802.

Franz MJ, VanWormer JJ, Crain AL, Boucher JL, Histon T, Caplan W, et al. 2007. "Weight loss outcomes: a systematic review and meta-analysis of weight-loss clinical trials with a minimum 1-year follow-up." *J Am Diet Assoc* 107: 1755–1767.

Freedman DS, Khan LK, Serdula MK, Dietz WH, Srinivasan SR, Berenson GS. 2005a. "Racial differences in the tracking of childhood BMI to adulthood." *Obes Res* 13: 928–935.

Freedman DS, Khan LK, Serdula MK, Dietz WH, Srinivasan SR, Berenson GS. 2005b. "The relation of childhood BMI to adult adiposity: the Bogalusa Heart Study." *Pediatrics* 115: 22–27.

Galani C, Schneider H. 2007. "Prevention and treatment of obesity with lifestyle interventions: review and meta-analysis." *Int J Public Health* 52: 348–359.

Gallo A. 1999. "Food advertising in the United States." In: Frazao E, ed. *America's eating habits: changes and consequences* (Agriculture Information Bulletin No. 750). Washington, DC: Economic Research Service/U.S. Department of Agriculture, 173–180. Available at: http://www.ers.usda.gov/publications/aib750/aib750i.pdf.

Healthy People Library Project. 2006. *Obesity: the science inside.* Washington, DC: American Association for the Advancement of Science.

Gantz W, Schwartz N, Angelini JR, Rideout V. 2007. *Food for thought: television food advertising to children in the United States.* Washington, DC: Kaiser Family Foundation.

Gardner CD, Kiazand A, Alhassan S, Kim S, Stafford RS, Balise RR, et al. 2007. "Comparison of the Atkins, Zone, Ornish, and LEARN diets for change in weight and related risk factors among overweight premenopausal women." *JAMA* 297: 969–977.

Giovannucci E, Ascherio A, Rimm EB, Colditz GA, Stampfer MJ, Willett WC. 1995. "Physical activity, obesity, and risk for colon cancer and adenoma in men." *Ann Intern Med* 122: 327–334.

GlaxoSmithKline. 2008. "alli: weight loss program for healthy weight loss." Available at: http://www.myalli.com. Accessed June 3, 2008.

Gortmaker SL, Must A, Perrin JM, Sobol AM, Dietz WH. 1993. "Social and economic consequences of overweight in adolescence and young adulthood." *New Engl J Med* 329: 1008–1012.

Gortmaker SL, Peterson K, Wiecha J, Sobol AM, Dixit S, Fox MK, et al. 1999. "Reducing obesity via a school-based interdisciplinary intervention among youth: Planet Health." *Arch Pediatr Adolesc Med* 153: 409–418.

Greves HM, Rivara FP. 2006. "Report card on school snack food policies among the United States' largest school districts in 2004–2005: room for improvement." *Int J Behav Nutr Phys Act* 3: 1.

Guo SS, Wu W, Chumlea WC, Roche AF. 2002. "Predicting overweight and obesity in adulthood from body mass index values in childhood and adolescence." *Am J Clin Nutr* 76: 653–658.

Hakim D, Confessore N. 2009, January 7. "Governor says New York is in a perilous situation." *New York Times.* Available at: http://www.nytimes.com/2009/01/08/nyregion/08state.html. Accessed January 23, 2009.

Hancox RJ. 2004. "Association between child and adolescent television viewing and adult health: a longitudinal birth cohort study." *Lancet* 364: 257–262.

Handy S, Clifton K. 2007. "Planning and the built environment: implications for obesity prevention." In: Kumanyika S, Brownson R, eds. *Handbook of obesity prevention: a resource for health professionals.* New York: Springer, 171–192.

Hawks SR. 2004. "Intuitive eating and the nutrition transition in Asia." *Asia Pac J Clin Nutr* 13: 194–203.

Hu FB. 2008. *Obesity epidemiology.* Oxford, UK: Oxford University Press.

Hu FB, Willett WC, Li T, Stampfer MJ, Colditz GA, Manson JE. 2004. "Adiposity as compared with physical activity in predicting mortality among women." *N Engl J Med* 351: 2694–2703.

Hubert HB, Feinleib M, McNamara PM, Castelli WP. 1983. "Obesity as an independent risk factor for cardiovascular disease: a 26-year follow-up of participants in the Framingham Heart Study." *Circulation* 67: 968–977.

Institute of Medicine of the National Academies of Science. 2002. *Dietary reference intakes for energy, carbohydrate, fiber, fat, fatty acids, cholesterol, protein, and amino acids (macronutrients)*. Washington, DC: National Academies Press.

International Agency for Research on Cancer/WHO. 2002. *IARC handbooks of cancer prevention: weight control and physical activity*. Vol 6. Lyon, France: Author.

James W, Jackson-Leach R, Mhurchu CN, Kalamara E, Shayeghi M, Rigby NJ, et al. 2003. "Overweight and obesity (high body mass index)." In: *Comparative quantification of health risks: global and regional burden of disease attributable to selected risk factors*. Geneva: World Health Organization, 497–596.

James WPT. 2008. "The fundamental drivers of the obesity epidemic." *Obes Rev* 9(Suppl 1): 6–13.

James WPT, Gill TP. 2008. "Prevention of obesity." In: Bray GA, Bouchard C, eds. *Handbook of obesity: clinical applications*. 3rd ed. New York: Informa Healthcare, 157–176.

Joos SK, Mueller WH, Hanis CL. 1984. "Diabetes alert study: weight history and upper body obesity in diabetic and non-diabetic Mexican American adults." *Ann Hum Biol* 11: 167–171.

Kaiser Family Foundation. 2004, February. *The role of media in childhood obesity* (Publ. No. 7030). Available at: http://www.kff.org.

Karlsson J, Taft C, Rydén A, Sjöström L, Sullivan M. 2007. "Ten-year trends in health-related quality of life after surgical and conventional treatment for severe obesity: the SOS Intervention Study." *Int J Obes* 31: 1248–1261.

Karlsson J, Taft C, Sjöström L, Torgerson JS, Sullivan M. 2003. "Psychosocial functioning in the obese before and after weight reduction: construct validity and responsiveness of the Obesity-Related Problems Scale." *Int J Obes* 27: 617–630.

Kimbro RT, Brooks-Gunn J, McLanahan S. 2007. "Racial and ethnic differentials in overweight and obesity among 3-year-old children." *Am J Public Health* 97: 298–305.

King GA, Fitzhugh EC, Bassett DR Jr, McLaughlin JE, Strath SJ, Swartz AM, et al. 2001. "Relationship of leisure-time physical activity and occupational activity to the prevalence of obesity." *Int J Obes Relat Metab Disord* 25: 606–612.

Kinnon JB. 2003, September. "At last! Etta James loses 200 pounds and finds a new zest for life." *Ebony*. Available at: http://findarticles.com/p/articles/mi_m1077/is_11_58/ai_106700554. Accessed May 30, 2008.

Klein S. 2004. "Clinical trial experience with fat-restricted vs carbohydrate restricted weight-loss diets." *Obes Res* 12(Suppl): 141–144.

Knowler WC, Barrett-Connor E, Fowler SE, Hamman RF, Lachin JM, Walker EA, et al. 2002. "Reduction in the incidence of type 2 diabetes with lifestyle intervention or metformin." *New Engl J Med* 13: 346–403.

Kolata G. 2002, April 16. "Asking if obesity is a disease or just a symptom." *New York Times*. Available at: http://www.nytimes.com/2002/04/16/health/16FAT.html.

Kramer RE, Daniels SR. 2008. "Special issues in treatment of pediatric obesity." In: Bray GA, Bouchard C, eds. *Handbook of obesity: clinical applications.* 3rd ed. New York: Informa Healthcare, 569–592.

Kumanyika S, Brownson RC. 2007. *Handbook of obesity prevention: a resource for health professionals.* New York: Springer.

Kung H-C, Hoyert DL, Xu J. 2008. "Deaths: final data for 2005." *Natl Vital Stat Rep* 56(10). Available at: http://www.cdc.gov/nchs/data/nvsr/nvsr56/nvsr56_10.pdf.

Kunkel D, Wilcox BL, Cantor J, Palmer E, Linn S, Dowrick P. 2004. "Psychological issues in the increasing commercialization of childhood." In: *Report of the American Psychological Association Task Force on Advertising and Children.* Washington, DC: APA.

Latifi R, Kellum J, De Maria E, Sugerman H. 2002. "Surgical treatment of obesity." In: Wadden TA, Stunkard AJ, eds. *Handbook of obesity treatment.* New York: Guilford, 339–356.

Lee C-D, Blair SN, Jackson AS. 1999. "Cardiorespiratory fitness, body composition, and all-cause and cardiovascular disease mortality in men." *Am J Clin Nutr* 69: 373–380.

Lee C-D, Jacobs DR, Schreiner PJ, Iribarren C, Hankinson A. 2007. "Abdominal obesity and coronary artery calcification in young adults: the Coronary Artery Risk Development in Young Adults (CARDIA) study." *Am J Clin Nutr* 86: 48–54.

Lee DC, Sui X, Church TS, Lee IM, Blair SN. 2009. "Associations of cardiorespiratory fitness and obesity on risks of impaired fasting glucose and type 2 diabetes in men." *Diabetes Care* 32: 257–262.

Lobstein T. "The prevention of obesity in childhood and adolescence." In: Bray GA, Bouchard C, eds. *Handbook of obesity: clinical applications.* 3rd ed. New York: Informa Healthcare, 131–156.

Loos RJ, Bouchard C. 2003. "Obesity—is it a genetic disorder?" *J Intern Med* 254: 401–425.

Lueck TJ, Severson K. 2006, December 6. "New York bans most trans fats in restaurants." *New York Times.* Available at: http://www.nytimes.com/2006/12/06/nyregion/06fat.html?_r=2. Accessed January 23, 2009.

Lutfiyya MN, Garcia R, Dankwa CM, Young T, Lipsky MS. 2008. "Overweight and obese prevalence rates in African American and Hispanic children: an analysis of data from the 2003–2004 National Survey of Children's Health." *J Am Board Fam Med* 21: 191–199.

Madanat HN, Brown RB, Hawks SR. 2007. "The impact of body mass index and Western advertising and media on eating style, body image and nutrition transition among Jordanian women." *Public Health Nutr* 10: 1039–1046.

Marshall SJ. 2004. "Relationships between media use, body fatness and physical activity in children and youth: a meta-analysis." *Int J Obes* 28: 1238–1246.

Martin DS. 2008. "'Wellness' a healthy investment for company." Available at: http://www.cnn.com/2008/HEALTH/diet.fitness/07/25/fn.healthy.company/index. html.

Mendez MA, Monteiro CA, Popkin BM. 2005. "Overweight exceeds underweight among women in most developing countries." Am J Clin Nutr 81:714–721.

Mendoza JA. 2007. "Television viewing, computer use, obesity, and adiposity in US preschool children." *Int J Behav Nutr Phys Act* 4: 44.

Must A, Jacques PF, Dallal GE, Bajema CJ, Dietz WH. 1992. "Long-term morbidity and mortality of overweight adolescents. A follow-up of the Harvard Growth Study of 1922 to 1935." N Engl J Med 327: 1350–1355.

National Center for Health Statistics. 2007. "Overweight, obesity, and healthy weight among persons 20 years of age and over, by sex, age, race and Hispanic origin, and poverty level: United States, 1960–1962 through 2001–2004." In: *Health, United States, 2007.* Available at: http://www.cdc.gov/nchs/data/hus/hus07.pdf#074.

National Heart, Lung, and Blood Institute. 2008. "What is asthma?" Available at: http://www.nhlbi.nih.gov/health/dci/Diseases/Asthma/Asthma_WhatIs.html. Accessed October 2008.

National Institute of Health. 2006. "Diabetes overview." Available at: http://diabetes. niddk.nih.gov/dm/pubs/overview/index.htm. Accessed October 2008.

Nielsen SJ, Popkin BM. 2004. "Changes in beverage intake between 1977 and 2001." *Am J Prev Med* 27: 205–210.

Ogden CL, Carroll MD, Curtin LR, McDowell MA, Tabak CJ, Flegal KM. 2006. "Prevalence of overweight and obesity in the United States, 1999–2004." JAMA 295: 1549–1555.

Ogden CL, Carroll MD, McDowell MA, FLegal KM. 2007. *Obesity among adults in the United States—no statistically significant change since 2003–2004* (NCHS Data Brief No. 1). Hyattsville, MD: National Center for Health Statistics.

Okholm D. 2000. "Rx for gluttony." *Christ Today* 44(10): 62. Available at: http://www.christianitytoday.com/ct/2000/september4/3.62.html?start=1.

Okie S. 2007. "New York to trans fats: you're out!" N Engl J Med 356: 2017–2021.

Okosun IS, Choi S, Matamoros T, Dever GE. 2001. "Obesity is associated with reduced self-rated general health status: evidence from a representative sample of White, Black, and Hispanic Americans." *Prev Med* 32: 429–436.

Olshansky SJ, Passaro DJ, Hershow RC, Layden J, Carnes BA, Brody J, et al. 2005. "A potential decline in life expectancy in the United States in the 21st century." N Engl J Med 352: 1138–1145.

Östman J, Britton M, Jonsson E. 2004. "Background." In: *Treating and preventing obesity: an evidence-based review.* Weinheim, Germany: Wiley-VCH, 15–29.

Patel SJ, Hu FB. 2008. "Short sleep duration and weight gain: A systematic review." Obesity 16: 643–653.

Parker S, Nichter M, Nichter M, Vuckovic N, Sims C, Ritenbaugh C. 1995. "Body image and weight concerns among African-American and white adolescent females: differences that make a difference." *Hum Organ* 54: 103–114.

Pereira MA, Kartashov AI, Ebbeling CB, Van Horn L, Slattery ML, Jacobs DR, et al. 2005. "Fast-food habits, weight gain, and insulin resistance (the CARDIA study): 15-year prospective analysis." *Lancet* 365: 36–42.

Peters LH. 1918. *Diet and health with key to calories.* Available at: http://books.google. com/books?id=-VORkj25YzsC&printsec=frontcover&dq=diet+and+health# PPA2,M1.

Petrelli JM, Calle EE, Rodriguez C, Thun MJ. 2002. "Body mass index, height, and postmenopausal breast cancer mortality in a prospective cohort of US women." *Cancer Causes Control* 13: 325–332.

Physical Activity Guidelines Advisory Committee. 2008. *Physical Activity Guidelines Advisory Committee report, 2008.* Washington, DC: U.S. Department of Health and Human Services.

Pietrobelli A, Espinoza MC, De Cristofaro P. 2008. "Childhood obesity: looking into the future." *Angiology* 59(Suppl 2): 30S–33S.

Pirozzo S, Summerbell C, Cameron C, Glasziou P. 2003. "Should we recommend low-fat diets for obesity?" *Obes Rev* 4(2): 83–90.

Popkin BM. 2003. "Dynamics of the nutrition transition toward the animal foods sector in China and its implications: a worried perspective." *J Nutr* 133: S3898–S3906.

Popkin BM. 2004. "The nutrition transition: an overview of world patterns of change." *Nutr Rev* 62(7): S140–S143.

Popkin BM. 2005. "Using research on the obesity pandemic as a guide to a unified vision of nutrition." *Public Health Nutr* 8: 724–729.

Popkin BM. 2007a. "Global context of obesity." In: Kumanyika S, Brownson R, eds. *Handbook of obesity prevention: a resource for health professionals.* New York: Springer, 227–238.

Popkin BM. 2007b. "Understanding global nutrition dynamics as a step towards controlling cancer incidence." *Nat Rev Cancer* 7: 61–67.

Popkin BM. 2008. "Will China's nutrition transition overwhelm its health care system and slow economic growth?" *Health Aff (Millwood)* 27: 1064–1076.

Raebel M, Malone DC, Conner DA, Xu S, Porter JA, Lanty FA. 2004. "Health services use and health care costs of obese and nonobese individuals." *Arch Intern Med* 164: 2135–2140.

Rand CS, Wright BA. 2000. "Continuity and change in the evaluation of ideal and acceptable body sizes across a wide age span." *Int J Eat Disord* 28: 90–100.

Resnicow K, Campbell MK, Carr C, McCarty F, Wang T, Periasamy S, et al. 2004. "Body and Soul: a dietary intervention conducted through African-American churches." *Am J Prev Med* 27: 97–105.

Reynolds SJ. 2007, July. "Star Jones Reynolds: 'I'm ready to open up.'" *Glamour.* Available at: http://www.glamour.com/health-fitness/2007/08/star-jones-weight. Accessed May 30, 2008.

Ritter M. 2005, March 9. "Shaq most obese in NBA? So says BMI." *NBC Sports.* Available at: http://nbcsports.msnbc.com/id/7129586. Accessed October 2008.

Rivera JA, Barquera S, González-Cossío T, Olaiz G, Sepúlveda J. 2004. "Nutrition transition in Mexico and other Latin American countries." *Nutr Rev* 62(7): S149–S157.

Rivera R. 2007, October 25. "New York reintroduces calorie rule." *New York Times.* Available at: http://www.nytimes.com/2007/10/25/nyregion/25calories.html. Accessed January 23, 2009.

Roker A. 2004a. "Weighing the risks (part 1): growing number of teens consider gastric bypass surgery." *Dateline.* Available at: http://www.msnbc.msn.com/id/6415459. Accessed May 30, 2008.

Roker A. 2004b. "Weighing the risks (part 2): complications." *Dateline.* Available at: http://www.msnbc.msn.com/id/6415560. Accessed May 30, 2008.

Roker A. 2004c. "Weighing the risks (part 3): Al's update." *Dateline.* Available at: http://www.msnbc.msn.com/id/6416184. Accessed May 30, 2008.

Roux L, Kuntz KM, Donaldson C, Goldie SJ. 2006. "Economic evaluation of weight loss intervention in overweight and obese women." *Obesity* 14: 1093–1106.

Rucker D, Padwal R, Li SK, Curioni C, Lau DC. 2007. "Long term pharmacotherapy for obesity and overweight: updated meta-analysis." *BMJ* 335: 1194–1199.

Runge CF. 2007. "Economic consequences of the obese." *Diabetes* 56: 2668–2672.

Ryan DH, Espeland MA, Foster GD, Haffner SM, Hubbard VS, Johnson KC, et al. 2003. "Look AHEAD (Action for Health in Diabetes): design and methods for a clinical trial of weight loss for the prevention of cardiovascular disease in type 2 diabetes." *Control Clin Trials* 24: 610–628.

Saul S. 2008, August 16. "Priced out of weight loss camp." *New York Times.* Available at: http://www.nytimes.com/2008/08/16/business/16camp.html?ref=health.

Schilling PL, Davis MM, Albanese CT, Dutta S, Morton J. 2008. "National trends in adolescent bariatric surgical procedures and implications for surgical centers of excellence." *J Am Coll Surg* 206: 1–12.

Schneider K, Green M, Neill M. 2004. "How to lose big." *People* 61(326). Available at: http://www.people.com/people/archive/article/0,,20149169,00.html. Accessed May 30, 2008.

Schneider M. 2007. "Media use and obesity in adolescent females." *Obesity* 15: 2328–2335.

Schwartz H. 1986. *Never satisfied: a cultural history of diets, fantasies and fat.* New York: The Free Press, 137.

Schwartz SM, Bansal VP, Hale C, Rossi M, Engle JP. 2008. "Compliance, behavior change, and weight loss with orlistat in an over-the-counter setting." *Obesity (Silver Spring)* 16: 623–629.

Sherwood NE, Jeffery RW, French SA, Hannan PJ, Murray DM. 2000. "Predictors of weight gain in the Pound of Prevention study." *Int J Obes Relat Metab Disord* 24: 395–403.

Shore SA. 2008. "Obesity and asthma: possible mechanisms." *J Allergy Clin Immunol* 121: 1087–1093; quiz 1094–1085.

Smith DE, Thompson JK, Raczynski JM, Hilner JE. 1999. "Body image among men and women in a biracial cohort: the CARDIA study." *Int J Eat Disord* 25: 71–82.

Solinas G, Vilcu C, Neels JG, Bandyopadhyay GK, Luo JL, Naugler W, et al. 2007. "JNK1 in hematopoietically derived cells contributes to diet-induced inflammation and insulin resistance without affecting obesity." *Cell Metab* 6: 386–397.

Stafford RS, Radley DC. 2003. "National trends in antiobesity medication use." *Arch Intern Med* 163: 1046–1050.

Stattin P, Lukanova A, Biessy C, Söderberg S, Palmqvist R, Kaaks R, et al. 2004. "Obesity and colon cancer: does leptin provide a link?" *Int J Cancer* 109: 149–152.

Steinbrook R. 2004. "Surgery for severe obesity." *N Engl J Med* 350: 1075–1079.

Steinhauer J. 2008, July 26. "California bars restaurant use of trans fats." *New York Times*. Available at: http://www.nytimes.com/2008/07/26/us/26fats.html?em. Accessed January 23, 2009.

Sugerman HJ, Sugerman EL, DeMaria EJ, Kellum JM, Kennedy C, Mowery Y, et al. 2003. "Bariatric surgery for severely obese adolescents." *J Gastrointest Surg* 7: 102–107; discussion 107–108.

Sullivan M, Karlsson J, Sjöström L, Backman L, Bengtsson C, Bouchard C, et al. 1993. "Swedish obese subjects (SOS)—an intervention study of obesity. Baseline evaluation of health and psychosocial functioning in the first 1743 subjects examined." *Int J Obes* 17: 503–512.

Swinburn B, Egger G. 2008. "Analyzing and influencing obesogenic environments." In: Bray GA, Bouchard C, eds. *Handbook of obesity: clinical applications*. 3rd ed. New York: Informa Healthcare, 177–194.

Swinburn B, Egger G, Raza F. 1999. "Dissecting obesogenic environments: the development and application of a framework for identifying and prioritizing environmental interventions for obesity." *Prev Med* 29: 563–570.

Teeple A. 2008, January 7. "Truth behind celebrities and weight loss surgery." Available at: http://www.docshop.com/2008/01/07/truth-behind-celebrities-and-weight-loss-surgery. Accessed May 30, 2008.

Thom T, Haase N, Rosamond W, Howard VJ, Rumsfeld J, Manolio T, et al. 2006. "Heart disease and stroke statistics—2006 update. A report from the American Heart Association Statistics Committee and Stroke Statistics Subcommittee." *Circulation* 113: e85–e151.

Thompson D, Edelsberg J, Colditz GA, Bird AP, Oster G. 1999. "Lifetime health and economic consequences of obesity." *Arch Intern Med* 159: 2177–2183.

Thompson D, Edelsberg J, Kinsey KL, Oster G. 1998. "Estimated economic cost of obesity to U.S. business." *Am J Health Promot* 13: 120–127.

Thompson OM, Yaroch AL, Moser RP, Petrelli JM, Smith-Warner SA, Masse LC, et al. 2008. "Fruit and vegetable knowledge of and adherence to recommendations: Results of the 2003 Health Information National Trends Survey (HINTS)." Unpublished data.

Thorpe KE, Florence CS, Howard DH, Joski P. 2004. "The impact of obesity on rising medical spending." *Health Aff (Millwood)* W4: 480–486.

Thygesen LC, Gronbaek M, Johansen C, Fuchs CS, Willett WC, Giovannucci E. 2008. "Prospective weight change and colon cancer risk in male US health professionals." *Int J Cancer* 123: 1160–1165.

Tsai WS, Inge TH, Burd RS. 2007. "Bariatric surgery in adolescents: recent national trends in use and in-hospital outcome." *Arch Pediatr Adolesc Med* 161: 217–221.

U.S. Department of Agriculture. n.d. "MyPyramid.gov: steps to a healthier you." Available at: http://www.mypyramid.gov.

U.S. Food and Drug Administration, Center for Drug Evaluation and Research. 1997. "FDA announces withdrawal of fenfluramine and dexfenfluramine (fen-phen)." Available at: http://www.fda.gov/CDER/news/phen/fenphenpr81597. Accessed September 12, 2008.

Vanwormer JJ, French SA, Pereira MA, Welsh EM. 2008. "The impact of regular self-weighing on weight management: a systematic literature review." *Int J Behav Nutr Phys Act* 5: 54.

Veuglers PJ, Fitzgerald AL. 2005. "Prevalence of and risk factors for childhood overweight and obesity." *CMAJ* 173: 607–613.

Wang G, Dietz WH. 2002. "Economic burden of obesity in youths aged 6 to 17 years: 1979–1999." *Pediatrics* 109: E81–81.

Wang LY, Yang Q, Lowry R, Wechsler H. 2003. "Economic analysis of a school-based obesity prevention program." *Obes Res* 11: 1313–1324.

Wang Y, Beydoun MA. 2007. "The obesity epidemic in the United States–Gender, age, socioeconomic, racial/ethnic, and geographic characteristics: A systematic review and meta-regression analysis." *Epidemiologic Reviews* 29: 6–28.

Wang Y, Beydoun MA, Liang L, Caballero B, Kumanyika SK. 2008. "Will all Americans become overweight or obese? Estimating the progression and cost of the US obesity epidemic." *Obesity (Silver Spring)* 16: 2323–2330.

Wang Y, Lobstein T. 2006. "Worldwide trends in childhood overweight and obesity." *Int J Pediatr Obes* 1: 11–25.

Wang Z, Zhai F, Du S, Popkin B. 2008. "Dynamic shifts in Chinese eating behaviors." *Asia Pac J Clin Nutr* 17: 123–130.

Wansink B, Kim J. 2005. "Bad popcorn in big buckets: portion size can influence intake as much as taste." *J Nutr Educ Behav* 37: 242–245.

Wansink B, Painter JE, North J. 2005. "Bottomless bowls: why visual cues of portion size may influence intake." *Obes Res* 13: 93–100.

Wardle J, Volz C, Golding C. 1995. "Social variation in attitudes to obesity in children." *Int J Obes Relat Metab Disord* 19: 562–569.

Wee CC, Phillips RS, Legedza ATR, Davis RB, Soukup JR, Colditz GA, Hamel MB. 2005. "Health care expenditures association with overweight and obesity among US adults: Importance of age and race." *AJPH* 95: 159–165.

Weinstein AR, Sesso HD, Lee IM, Rexrode KM, Cook NR, Manson JE, et al. 2008. "The joint effects of physical activity and body mass index on coronary heart disease risk in women." *Arch Intern Med* 168: 884–890.

Weller WE, Hannan EL. 2006. "Relationship between provider volume and postoperative complications for bariatric procedures in New York State." *J Am Coll Surg* 202: 753–761.

Westphal SA. 2008. "Obesity, abdominal obesity, and insulin resistance." *Clin Cornerstone* 9: 23–31.

Whitney EN, Rolfes SR. 1996. *Understanding nutrition*. 7th ed. Minneapolis/St. Paul: West Publishing.

Whorton JC. 1982. *Crusaders for fitness: the history of American health reformers*. Princeton, NJ: Princeton University Press.

Wiecha JL, Peterson KE, Ludwig DS, Kim J, Sobol A, Gortmaker SL. 2006. "When children eat what they watch: impact of television viewing on dietary intake in youth." *Arch Pediatr Adolesc Med* 160: 436–442.

Wikipedia. n.d. "Lane Bryant." Available at: http://en.wikipedia.org/wiki/Lane_Bryant.

Wikipedia. n.d. "Mother goddess." Available at: http://en.wikipedia.org/wiki/Mother_Goddess.

Willett WC, Hu FB, Colditz GA, Manson JE. 2005. "Underweight, overweight, obesity, and excess deaths." JAMA 294: 551; author reply 552–553.

Willett WC, Manson JE, Stampfer MJ, Colditz GA, Rosner B, Speizer FE, et al. 1995. "Weight, weight change, and coronary heart disease in women. Risk within the 'normal' weight range." JAMA 273: 461–465.

Williamson DA, Womble LG, Zucker NL, Reas DL, White MA, Blouin DC, et al. 2000. "Body image assessment for obesity (BIA-O): development of a new procedure." *Int J Obes* 24: 1326–1332.

Wing R. 2008. "Behavioral approaches to the treatment of obesity." In: Bray GA, Bouchard C, eds. *Handbook of obesity: clinical applications*. 3rd ed. New York: Informa Healthcare, 227–248.

Wing R, Hill JO. 2001. "Successful weight loss maintenance." *Annu Rev Nutr* 21: 323–341.

Wing R, Phelan S. 2005. "Long-term weight loss maintenance." *Am J Clin Nutr* 82(Suppl): 222S–225S.

Wolf AM, Colditz GA. 1994. "The cost of obesity: the US perspective." *Pharmacoeconomics* 5(Suppl 1): 34–37.

Wolf AM, Colditz GA. 1996. "Social and economic effects of body weight in the United States." *Am J Clin Nutr* 63(Suppl): 466S–469S.

Wolf AM, Colditz GA. 1998. "Current estimates of the economic cost of obesity in the United States." *Obes Res* 6: 97–106.

Wolf AM, Finer N, Allshouse AA, Pendergast KB, Sherrill BH, Caterson I, et al. 2008. "PROCEED: Prospective Obesity-Cohort of Economic Evaluation and Determinants: baseline health and healthcare utilization of the US sample." *Diabetes Obes Metab* 10: 1248–1260.

Wolin KY, Colditz GA. 2008. "Can weight loss prevent cancer?" *Br J Cancer* 99: 995–999.

World Cancer Research Fund/American Institute for Cancer Research. 2007. *Food, nutrition, physical activity, and the prevention of cancer: a global perspective.* Washington, DC:. Available at: http://www.dietandcancerreport.org.

World Health Organization. 2005. "Preventing chronic diseases: a vital investment: WHO global report." Available at: http://www.who.int/chp/chronic_disease_report/full_report.pdf. Accessed November 2008.

Writing Group for the SEARCH for Diabetes in Youth Study. 2007. "Incidence of diabetes in youth in the United States." *JAMA* 297: 2716–2724.

Yang Z, Hall AG. 2008. "The financial burden of overweight and obesity among elderly Americans: the dynamics of weight, longevity, and health care cost." *Health Serv Res* 43: 849–868.

Young LR, Nestle M. 2002. "The contribution of expanding portion sizes to the US obesity epidemic." *Am J Public Health* 92: 246–249.

Young LR, Nestle M. 2003. "Expanding portion sizes in the US marketplace: implications for nutrition counseling." *J Am Diet Assoc* 103: 231–234.

Yum Brands. 2009. "Yum! China." Available at: http://www.yum.com/company/china.asp. Accessed April 2009.

Zhang C, Rexrode KM, van Dam RM, Li TY, Hu FB. 2008. "Abdominal obesity and the risk of all-cause, cardiovascular, and cancer mortality: sixteen years of follow-up in US women." *Circulation* 117: 1658–1667.

Zinzindohoue F, Chevallier JM, Douard R, Elian N, Ferraz JM, Blanche JP, et al. 2003. "Laparoscopic gastric banding: a minimally invasive surgical treatment for morbid obesity: prospective study of 500 consecutive patients." *Ann Surg* 237: 1–9.

Index

About the Authors

KATHLEEN Y. WOLIN, Sc.D., is Assistant professor of surgery at the Washington University School of Medicine in St. Louis, MO, where she is also a member of the Siteman Cancer Center and an Institute for Public Health Scholar. Dr. Wolin has authored numerous publications on obesity and physical activity and conducts research on the role of both in cancer prevention and control.

JENNIFER M. PETRELLI is an independent science writer with master's degrees in both epidemiology and nutrition. Ms. Petrelli has co-authored several peer reviewed papers in the area of cancer research.